How to Live to be **100** in Spite of Your Doctor

How to Live to be **100** in Spite of Your Doctor

Add years to your life and life to your years!

Dr. Bruce C. Hagen

The Hagen Publishing Company
Sioux Falls, South Dakota

Produced and distributed by
The Hagen Publishing Company
1300 W. Murphy Drive
Sioux Falls, SD 57108
ISBN 0-9778763-0-6

Printed in the United States of America
Editorial assistance provided by Griffith Publishing,
Boise, Idaho
Cover design by Linda Griffith, Portland, Oregon

Websites:
www.DRBRUCEHAGEN.COM
www.HOWTOLIVETOBE100INSPITEOFYOURDOCTOR.COM

Dedication

To my wife Bethel Mae Hagen for being my inspiration, for putting up with my foibles, for believing in me before my own relatives did, for being the perfect mother of our six children, and for being my number one patient.

To our six children, Dr. Bruce Jon, Dr. Dan, Dr. Mark Palmer, Eric William Hagen, esq., and to our two beautiful daughters Lisa and Lori who are living proof that Darwin was wrong when he said "Like produces like."

To all of our children and grandchildren for their brains, beauty, performance, athleticism, in the classroom, and in their churches.

Disclaimer

The information contained in this book has been
gleaned from a variety of sources over the past fifty-
five years and while I have selected facts and opinions
from sources I consider to be reliable, they cannot be
validated by myself as absolutely accurate in all
respects. The book is for the reader's personal interest
and should not be considered a medical guide. Consult
with your personal care provider for advice related to
your situation.

Contents

Watch what you eat 76

A word about chiropractic 161

Appendix 177

Recommended reading 179

Recommended subscriptions 180

Curriculum Vitae: Bruce C. Hagen 181

Introduction

Why was this book written? What right do I have to write a book about living to be 100?

Joyce Griffith, who assisted me in finishing this book, calls this "The Doctor Bashing Book." Let me unequivocally state that is not my intent. Everyone recognizes the value of traditional medical care especially when trauma is involved.

Unfortunately, the paradigm of medicine is fraught with danger. First of all a proper diagnosis must be made and is likely to be in error. Drugs are prescribed that have potentially dangerous side effects. Wrong dosages are often prescribed.

A combination of several different drugs may interact. If surgery is utilized, mistakes are frequently made. Hospital infections are ubiquitous. Nurses are overburdened. Proper instructions for prescriptions and home care are not carried out.

Forty percent of all the drugs prescribed may never be taken by the patient. (That may not be all that bad). The FDA frequently approves drugs that cause more harm than good and are slow to remove them after deaths occur from their use. Medical training is subsidized by drug companies who expect the new doctors to recommend their products. Nearly $40,000 in advertising in medical journals is spent per doctor per year extolling the benefits and minimizing the adverse effects of their products. And oftentimes alternative therapies might have been more productive for the patient but were never offered as an option. The tremendous cost of medical care often bankrupts the patient.

Twenty-four of the top twenty-five lobbying interests in Washington are health care related. When Medicare was enacted in 1965 the AMA spent $300 million lobbying against it and when they realized it was going to pass jumped on the band wagon and kicked out the care that was supposed to be provided by chiropractors, optometrists, podiatrists, physical therapists, dentists, and drugs.

Medicare was supposed to cost seven billion dollars per year. Today it costs more than thirty times that much.

The Supreme Court of the United States found the AMA guilty of Antitrust violations in 1988 by conspiring to eliminate the chiropractic profession.

Chiropractors are now serving as commissioned officers in our armed services, veterans' hospitals, in many private and municipal hospitals. Almost every professional sports teams have chiropractors treating injuries and enhancing the performance of their athletes.

Most Americans are over medicated, excessive surgeries are performed, and we've never been sicker. According to Dr. Lorraine Day, Americans rank behind more than seventy nations in the status of health care in the world. The only first place category in the health care field that we Americans rank number one is in expenditures. Although we are only five percent of the world's population we consume fifty percent of all the drugs that are consumed in the world.

Most doctors have little knowledge of nutrition and its vital role in healing their patients. Eighty percent of doctors have little knowledge in the value of chiropractic care, massage therapy, nutrition, and acupuncture.

If a doctor embraces therapies outside the mainstream of medicine he is often ostracized by his profession, and his license may be in jeopardy.

During the past fifty-five years I've not missed a single day of work. My wife of fifty-three years has never taken a prescription drug. For more than fifty years I did not find it necessary to take either prescription or over-the-counter drugs. Our six children never had a pediatrician. They had excellent attendance records, excelled in athletics and intellectual achievements.

I've treated 50,000 patients from almost every state and province of Canada and several foreign countries. Many came to our clinics on crutches, in wheel chairs, on disability, and living on drugs. My sons and I treated almost fifty employees of a major meat packing company who were advised by MDs, chiropractors, and physical therapists to have back or carpal tunnel surgery. None of the patients we treated wound up in surgery. One patient, who had exprienced two back surgeries and had not worked for five years, was returned to work in four months pain free.

I've authored the largest nutritional chart ever published as well as a Depletions Chart that illustrates what nutrients you lose from taking aspirin, alcohol, antacids, caffeine, antibiotics, birth control pills, cholesterol drugs, cola drinks, diuretics, estrogen, laxatives, steroids, and sugar, or from smoking or excessive stress. I've treated hundreds of athletes without surgery or drugs and enhanced their athletic performance.

At age 76 I'm still working ten to sixteen hours a day and enjoying every minute of it. I play tennis every morning and golf three times each week and practice three days each week treating patients in our clinics in Sioux Falls, South Dakota and Council Bluffs, Iowa. My wife Beth also looks young and is often assumed to be married to one of my sons when they're seen together. Although all males on both sides of my family are bald in their twenties, I still have a nearly full head of hair. I do take a lot of vitamins.

For more than fifty years I've saved health articles, attended seminars and classes at major universities and clinics, been trained in non-medical treatment protocols, and tried all kinds of natural therapies. Some worked. Some didn't. One article I saved from the *Davenport Times* stated in 1952 that no one would ever suffer with arthritis again. A new drug called Cortisone would cure everyone.

There is no miracle cure, no single item that can guarantee life and vitality. There is a common-sense way of thinking that I have attempted to depict in this book. It is based on what I've learned through the years and the knowledge I have gained that I believe can be of value to others who want to add life to their years.

Because of factors we've inherited, mistakes we made earlier in our lives, or unfortunate circumstances we've encountered along the way, you and I may not live to be 100.

That is all past. Today is the first day of the rest of our lives. Let's live this day and every day that follows with determination to enjoy life and good health to 100 and beyond. It's up to us.

The sad state of health care today

The state of health care in America is abysmal.

America is one of the best countries in the world to be treated for trauma but one of the worst to seek treatment of acute and chronic diseases.

Many senior citizens my age have undergone bypass surgery or have had a stent installed, even though a Pritikin Diet and Exercise Program could have prevented eighty percent of those operations.

Diabetes is a growing problem in America. Obesity affects two-thirds of our adult population and one-third of our adolescent population. The incidence of obesity has doubled in the past twenty years. This trend in obesity is already affecting life expectancy tables.

According to Robert Mendelson, M.D., when doctors go on strike and refuse to treat the general public the death rate generally goes down—by as much as fifty percent. In his book *Confessions of a Medical Heretic* he states that a permanent strike by doctors would be good for health care.

Everyone is concerned about AIDS. Sixteen thousand people die each year from AIDS. Sixteen thousand people also die each year from pain killing drugs, NSAIDs. Which problems get the most publicity and funds?

Health care systems profit from disease, not health. Americans spend almost two trillion dollars annually on health care. That comes to almost $6,000 per person for medical services. Even at that high level of spending, Americans have a higher percentage of cancer, heart disease, diabetes, migraines, arthritis, strokes, high blood pressure, ulcers, back surgeries, hysterectomies, gall bladder surgeries and iatrogenesis (doctor-caused diseases or death) than do the residents of any other country in the world.

The United States has the highest death rate from asthma and the highest rate of infection from hepatitis B. According to Dr. Joseph Mercola (www.mercola.com), the health care system "is crumbling before our eyes. Our country cannot afford this nightmare mess." This is said even as health care spending continues to grow faster than the economy and is expected to reach $3 trillion by 2020.

No wonder twenty million American families had trouble paying their medical bills last year. A study reporting this was released June 30, 2004, by the Center for Studying Health Care System Change. Two thirds of the twenty million people with problems paying their medical bills did not have health insurance. NBC Nightly News reported that 800,000 people file for bankruptcy each year due to high medical bills.

Medical doctors are great for treating trauma and eye disorders, but in general the practice of medicine in all of its aspects is both expensive and dangerous.

I once read a doctor's statement that if the patient lived the doctor saved his life. If he died the Lord called him home. After fifty-five years of treating the sick I'm convinced there are very few miracles in medicine. Many times after an autopsy is preformed even the doctor is astonished at what kept the patient alive.

The reality is that if there are problems, they could be the result of bad medical practice. According to a new book written by two PhDs and two medical doctors, the leading cause of death in America is doctor-caused. The book, *Death by Medicine,* reports that according to mortality studies by all of the various specialties in medicine that 768,000 deaths occur each year from medical treatments, hospital infections, unnecessary surgeries, drug reactions, failure to diagnose, neglect, inappropriate treatment, wrong dosages, and drugs that never should have been put on the market.

Americans spend more money on health care than any other nation in the world. The expenditures are approaching 16 percent of our Gross National Product.

Former senator Tom Daschle recently reported that the average Medicare patient receives seventeen prescriptions per year.

That's enough medicine to make them really sick. I've talked to patients who were taking fifty-five pills per day. The world's smartest chemist would be unable to predict the toxic side effects of that much medication.

The University of Arizona School of Pharmacy reported in 2001 that Americans spend seventy-five billion dollars each year on drugs and seventy-six billion dollars each year treating the side effect of those drugs.

I cannot name a single chronic disease that medicine has conquered in the last fifty years. The medical press states that we are conquering cancer, but we've had a three-fold increase in mortality from cancer since 1950. Fifty years ago less than ten percent of the population died of cancer. Now thirty percent of our population dies of cancer. Yet almost daily we read medical propaganda of how medicine is curing cancer. I cannot think of a worse diagnosis today than telling a patient he or she has cancer.

The *World Factbook* shows that the people of sixty nations live as long or longer than Americans when in comes to life expectancy at birth (2005 est.). The Geography IQ of the World Atlas ranks infant mortality in America as thirty sixth in the world. However, last year infant mortality increased in the US so now we rank fortieth. A baby born in the cane fields of Cuba has a better chance of survival than one born in an American hospital.

While attending a Health Systems Management course at the Harvard School of Public Health in the 1990s I was privileged to sit next to the Minister of Health from Iceland. He had designed a birthing complex of five birthing stations next to a surgical center. Most babies born in Iceland are delivered by midwives. When complications arise they are moved into the surgical center. Their infant mortality is much lower than ours.

Americans have the highest incidence of Caesarian born babies in the world. Each Caesarian delivery involves a whole set of complications, many of them life-threatening.

Another problem in birthing is the common practice of inducing labor so that the delivery will take place at a more convenient time for the doctor. It may fit the doctor's schedule better, but the facts are that interfering with Mother Nature brings on more complications.

One study of 1,000 newborns found that three out of four newly born babies have neurological damage caused by delivery.

Eighty pounds of pressure may be exerted on the head and neck of a newborn during delivery.

A million-dollar diagnosis

Medical science has produced some spectacular diagnostic instruments in the past twenty-five years. A colleague of mine observes that you can spend a million dollars for a diagnosis, but you can't spend a nickel to cure your disease.

CT Scans, MRIs, endoscopic surgeries, bone scans, and DNA testing are just a few of the many scientific achievements in diagnostic medicine. Unfortunately, the treatment of diseases has not kept parallel with the discovery of new technology for diagnosing them.

A young friend I'll call Brianna was being treated for a skin condition. The parents finally decided to go to a state university hospital. I called the parents after they returned to see how Brianna had done.

"The diagnostic services were wonderful," the father said. "They looked in her mouth and her anus and did all kinds of blood tests, urine tests, and much more. I am totally pleased with our visit to this diagnostic center."

"Has she improved?" I asked. "Is her skin responding to the treatment?"

"She's no better than she was before she went to the diagnostic center," he said, "but I am so pleased that we took her there."

Too many errors

Medical science is predicated on the establishment of a proper diagnosis so that the physician can treat the patient. Unfortunately, there are many vagaries in the diagnosis of disease. Two major studies at Harvard School of Medicine and the Mayo Clinic many years ago found that medical diagnoses based on autopsy findings were in error fifty percent of the time.

In other words, after a patient visited these outstanding medical centers, a diagnosis was made and then the patient died. They did an autopsy and compared the autopsy findings with the medical diagnosis of record. They found that they were in error fifty percent of the time.

The degree of diagnostic accuracy varied with certain conditions.

> **HOW TO FIND A DOCTOR**
>
> Patients frequently tell me they have trouble finding a doctor. I ask them where they call for a doctor. They tell me they try to call his home (chances are he has an unlisted number), his office, or the hospital. No wonder they can't find the doctor. All they have to do is call his country club, his investment broker or his farm.

If the diagnosis is inaccurate fifty percent of the time at the Mayo Clinic and the Harvard School of Medicine, what is it like in Podunk where the doctor spends five minutes with the patient, fails to run an MRI, CT Scan, or elaborate blood test, and makes a snap diagnosis? In order for the doctor to treat you properly, the diagnosis must be correct. After the diagnosis is made, the doctor has to determine which one of 5,000 medications to prescribe for it or which treatment protocol to utilize. The dosage for a 15-pound baby would be entirely different from that for a 300-pound adult. The prescription for a one-year-old infant may be entirely different than for an 80-year-old patient. One patient's body chemistry may be entirely different from another patient's.

Add to this the factor of a combative effect of patients taking the combination of several drugs. Will the latest prescription enhance the recovery process or have a deleterious effect upon the patient?

Medical errors account for over 100,000 deaths per year according to the *Journal of the American Medical Association.* The author thinks this is the tip of the iceberg because many patients have fatal outcomes that are not reported properly because of the doctors' fear of malpractice lawsuits.

It amazes me when surviving relatives of patients that have expired place ads in the local papers thanking the doctors and the hospital for their wonderful care. Hey, buddy, your relative died!

Health care systems

One system we have in the U.S. for delivering medical care is called Managed Health Care. The idea is that a lot of people will be taken care of by several doctors, and because most of the people are healthy, the cost of caring for those who are sick will be much lower than with traditional insurance plans.

I have to ask this question: What good is Managed Health Care if it doesn't allow you to see the doctor that can help you with your problem? Many people today are more concerned about getting reimbursed rather than getting well. Doctors, hospitals, and drug companies have gotten richer, and patients have become poorer.

At our clinic we are providers for several health care plans. If, however, someone comes to our office who is not a member of one of our health care plans, we don't let that stop us from helping that person get well. We have special plans for patients without insurance coverage or whose plan does not include us as providers.

When Dr. T. H. Pluess convinced me to become a doctor, he told me a story about Henry Ford, the man who designed and built the first Cadillac automobile. He soon realized that very few people could afford a luxury car like the Cadillac. His goal in life was to build an automobile that everyone in America could afford to own. Henry Ford accomplished his goal. Dr. Pluess went on to say he wanted to render health services that every patient could afford.

> The six most dangerous words in the world of health care are "I thought it would go away."

We like that philosophy. Our staff at the Hagen Clinics believes that a proper fee is one that's charged and paid without gloom on either side. For most patients the care costs them hardly anything because Medicare, group insurance, HMO, car accident insurance, workers' compensation, and self-insurance cover most of our patients. If a patient of ours is concerned about charges we always try to answer any questions before we begin the care.

Remember that the six most dangerous words in the world of health care are "I thought it would go away." On the other hand, with socialized medicine, the prolonged wait for medical services is so long that patients often recover on their own without the doctors interfering with their normal recovery.

I remember seeing a headline in a national publication years ago stating, "The patient died without medical assistance."

Sir William Osler, famed founder of the John Hopkins Medical School in Baltimore, Maryland pontificated that "to interfere with Nature's efforts to heal disease costs too much money, too much time, too much in suffering, and the prolongation of illness, far too much on the whole, for Nature knows how to cure disease but man does not, and anything that could not be cured by Nature must forever remain uncured." Osler also stated that he could count on the fingers of one hand without repeating all of the so-called remedies that were of any use to the human race. Not long before he died he said, "The cause of disease is a great mystery."

Voltaire said, "We put medicine, of which we know little, into bodies about which we know less to cure diseases of which we know nothing at all."

Living longer and better is still possible

During the past fifty-five years I've never missed a day of work due to sickness and have never taken an aspirin, a Tylenol tablet, or an ibuprofen product—and never needed Viagra. I've treated over 50,000 patients naturally without drugs or surgery.

My greatest claim to fame is the fact that I originated the slogan, "Thank you for not smoking." Another accomplishment was made as a student studying for my doctorate. I authored the most complete nutritional chart ever published. I updated it in 1981, 1983, 2000, and again in 2004. It's now five times as large as it was in 1952.

A voracious reader of health care information, I've passed that information on to my patients. I've spent over $100,000 visiting outstanding health care clinics and attending seminars. I've studied and treated patients in Japan, Russia, Australia, England, Canada, Mexico and the Caribbean. I've lectured to doctors of every state in the USA and all the provinces of Canada, Poland, and Russia.

My conclusion: The state of health care in America is pathetic. We spend almost twice as much per person on health care as countries in the rest of the world. Yet the people of more than sixty nations live longer than we do and we rank below more than thirty-six nations on infant mortality. Here are more facts to support my claim:

- Two thirds of our adult population is obese, and many of our children are destined to decades of ill health due to the wrong diet and lack of exercise.

- Eighty percent of our lifetime health care costs occur in the last year of our life.

- Some doctors believe that every patient that leaves his or her office needs to have a new prescription in hand. The side effects of even three or four different drugs are absolutely unpredictable.

- We have five times as many back surgeries and hysterectomies in the U.S. as in Europe.

- Can you name one disease that can be cured by medicine? My mentor, Dr. T. H. Pluess, told me 55 years ago there wasn't a cure in a carload of medicine.

- Ninety percent of all medicines are palliative and not curative. They numb your brain so you can't feel your pain. They either speed something up or slow something down. They don't normalize body functions.

- Receiving a flu shot for five years in a row after age 55 increases your risk of Alzheimer's disease tenfold, according to the Blaylock Wellness Report Vol. 3, No 2.

Avoid doctors (and hospitals)

This might seem like strange advice in a book by a doctor, but I know, and you will soon find out, that avoiding doctors is a good idea.

Of course I don't recommend doing your own heart surgery or writing your own prescriptions to get the medicine you need. Doctors with traditional medical training and experience can be very helpful at times. I've just found that people who stay away from doctors are a lot healthier than those who are always making another appointment to see the family doctor.

I'm not a traditional doctor. I'm a chiropractor. As I explained in the last chapter I don't consider illness and treatment the same way that doctors do after they go through the usual seven to ten years of post-college medical training.

This book doesn't represent the opinions of all chiropractors, of course, but when you finish reading these pages you should have a pretty good idea about what many chiropractors believe and practice in their work of healing.

A few years ago Arnold Schwartzenegger was quoted in the magazine, *Dynamic Chiropractic,* saying "Chiropractic is about natural, preventive health care. What you are doing, and I have experienced this for the last thirty years myself on my own body, means that whenever I have a problem...I go to a chiropractor, and my problems are gone in no time."

I've traveled with chiropractic teams to Jamaica, Ukraine, and Poland. We have given more than a million dollars' worth of chiropractic services to the patients we have met on these trips as well as thousands of pairs of shoes and tons of vitamins, clothing, and dental supplies.

I remember seeing Rodney, a patient at my chiropractic clinic who had been injured in a meat packing plant in Iowa and had back surgery. Two years later he was still suffering from pain and immobility, so he had his second back surgery. It made him worse. For the next three years he was disabled. His wife hid his guns and pills from him because he was suffering from such horrible pain that he was considering taking his life. He heard about my clinic, and he and his wife drove the ninety miles to the city where my clinic was located. Rodney was lying on a mattress in back of their station wagon. They pulled into a filling station for directions.

"You're going to the Hagen Clinic?" the attendant asked. "You might as well go home. He'll never help you."

After four days of adjustments every morning and afternoon, Rodney was off all pain medications, and four months later he went back to work. The safety manager at the meat packing company called my clinic and made arrangements to send nearly fifty employees who were destined to have back or carpal tunnel surgery to see me. No patient that was treated ended up having surgery.

Rodney stopped by the filling station to scold the attendant for almost keeping him from being a patient at the Hagen Clinic. The attendant apologized. Later he became a patient at the clinic.

Stay away from doctors if you can

My life insurance agent recently told me that his doctor advised him, "If you want to live a long life, stay away from doctors." Several members of my family would have been well served if they had heeded that advice.

My oldest sister had a pain in her side. They told her it was appendicitis and removed her appendix. She still had the pain. They said it must be gall bladder trouble, so they removed her gall bladder. The pain persisted. Then their diagnosis was, "You must have an ulcer," so they planned to remove a major portion of her stomach.

When they opened her abdomen they found she had an abdominal aneurysm.

Instead of calling in a cardiovascular surgeon and installing a Dacron tube, they removed three-fifths of her stomach. She had a total of 151 blood transfusions and died at the age of 32. Had I not told hospital authorities that I was a doctor and wanted to see her records we would never have known the facts in her case.

My cousin Jim was the same age as I am. They gave him so many powerful drugs for his asthma that they ruined his kidneys. He wound up on dialysis.

One day they got an air bubble in his blood stream during his dialysis treatment and lost him. He was only 43 years old.

Jim's sister-in-law was advised to have a flu shot. She complied with her doctor's wishes. She's still in a wheelchair from her reaction to that flu shot.

As youngsters growing up in Wisconsin, the kids in our family didn't have a personal physician. I only saw a doctor twice in my first seventeen years of life. Once was to have my tonsils out. I can still smell the ether on the cloth they put over my face. My dad never paid the doctor, which served him right for taking out a healthy organ.

On two occasions when I cut my foot the local policeman sewed me up.

When I enlisted in the USAF twenty-four days before World War II was officially declared over, I thought, "Great! Now I can have all those life-saving vaccines that I couldn't afford as a child." After the smallpox shot I wound up in the military hospital with a shoulder that festered for one year. The hospital was full of young men suffering from reactions to vaccinations. I still have a spur on that shoulder that I'm positive came from that vaccine.

After basic training I was sent to Guam. They decided to give all of us a flu shot. The next day I felt like I had been run over by a two-ton truck. My buddies carried me up to the dispensary. They pricked my finger with a nail because they couldn't find a needle. The blood test told them I had the flu and they advised me that I needed a flu shot. I told them "No thank you." That's what made me sick in the first place.

Before I was discharged from the Air Force I went down to the dispensary and insisted that they bring my shot record up to date. Years later I discovered that many times vaccines kill more people than they save. I'll deal with vaccines at greater length in a later chapter. Back to family stories.

My cousin is a minister, now retired. For many years he worked as a chaplain in a large nursing home. He told me on numerous occasions doctors would tell the head nurse that there was no hope for Mary or Joe.

They would advise them to take all of their medicines away from them and let them die. Ironically, several of those patients recovered after their meds were taken away.

My father-in-law broke his back when he pushed my sister-in-law out from under a falling farm elevator and the elevator landed on top of him. They had to dig him out from under the machine. Arthritis eventually settled in his spine. He wound up in the hospital from all the medicines he was taking. His medicines were causing all kinds of problems. He left the hospital and went to a chiropractor every day for twenty-eight days.

When he was over eighty years old, he worked cutting down trees in below zero weather. He continued to see his chiropractor every two weeks for several years. When he turned 86 the Iowa Highway Patrol told him he could only drive within a 25-mile radius of his home.

After he hadn't seen his chiropractor for almost a year, he went to the local physician, who prescribed a fluid pill. The fluid pill washed the potassium out of his system, so they gave him Slow-K. That irritated his stomach so they gave him Maalox. That caused him to be constipated. So they gave him a laxative.

I sat down with him one day, and he lined his pills up on the kitchen table. Because he took the fluid pill he was now taking fourteen other medicines.

He eventually got so sick and weak that he finally agreed to go to the nursing home in the neighboring town. The doctor in that town took away all of his medicines. He recovered remarkably well, and it looked like he would be able to return home. Then the doctor decided to give him a new medicine. He died thirty minutes after taking it.

My mother-in-law lived to be ninety years of age. She lived in a three-story house. I think running up and down those steps added to her longevity.

We family members were worried that she might fall and wouldn't be discovered for several hours or days. She chose to go to an assisted living facility. During her first month there she fell and broke her hip when getting out of a chair. My wife went back home to be with her in the hospital and was concerned that her mother's skin was very dark under her eyes. Having attended nurses training after high school, she advised the head nurse that her mother needed a blood test. The nurse told my wife she couldn't order a test because her doctor was on vacation. When he returned, the blood test showed she was extremely low in sodium (most people have too much).

They started to give her sodium directly into her veins. She suffered a myocardial infarction and died. I think they gave her too much sodium too fast.

My sister's husband had chest pain. His cholesterol level was over 600.

They decided to do a heart catheterization. He died on the table. I don't think it's a very good idea to run a tube up a blood vessel when you have a 600 cholesterol level. He died the day before his wedding anniversary.

During my wife's first pregnancy her ankles were swollen about two weeks before she gave birth to our oldest son. The doctor gave her a prescription for Stilbestrol, a drug that causes abortions in cattle. She never filled the prescription. We treated her naturally and her swelling went away. When the doctor examined her in the delivery room he commented how the Stilbestrol had taken away the swelling.

Several years later scientists discovered that women who were given Stilbestrol had offspring with vaginal and testicular cancers.

My daughter-in-law worked for a factory in Sioux City, Iowa. She developed carpal tunnel syndrome. Her company sent her to a local orthopedic surgeon who performed an EMG. Before he got the results of the EMG he operated on her hand. He operated to release the wrong nerve. He advised her to have the operation done again. She requested that she be given a general anesthetic instead of a local one. After they gave her an injection they started to paint her knees.

She told them she was there for carpal tunnel surgery. They ignored her until she screamed at them. They then discovered the next patient was the one who was supposed to have knee surgery.

The surgery failed to relieve her symptoms. They somehow convinced her to do the other hand.

Her three carpal tunnel surgeries left her totally disabled and on Medicare at twenty-five years of age. She dropped her infant son causing physical damage to him because of the weakness caused by the surgeries. After a severe whiplash accident she consulted with my son, a chiropractor. He did her so much good that she married him.

The purpose of this book is to help you prevent health problems like those my family members have suffered and to prevent surgery whenever possible.

In the 'nick of time'

I'm skeptical about traditional medicine after fifty years of watching doctors ride the glory train of healing without deserving the praise—or the pay.

Over the course of fifty years treating 50,000 patients from all walks of life, I have discovered that everybody who has had their appendix out has been told it was done "just in the nick of time."

A number of years ago, a midwestern school of medicine examined thirty-three appendices removed from various patients. They did pathology studies and found that two of the thirty-three were inflamed; the rest were healthy.

John, one of my favorite patients, was at the hospital while my wife was delivering our first child. I asked him what he was doing there.

"I'm waiting for my daughter," John said. "Her doctors said she was having an attack of appendicitis, and they wanted to remove it."

I listened as he continued his tale.

"I insisted that she drive home and have it removed at home at the local doctor's hospital," John said. "By the time she'd arrived at home, her pain was gone. They did a white count and said that it was up to 9,000, and she needed her appendix removed." (By the way, 7,000 to 10,000 is the normal white blood cell count.)

"John," I said, "when the doctor comes down from operating, he is going to tell you, 'I got it just in the nick of time.' "

A few minutes after our conversation, the doctor came down the steps with his stethoscope around his neck and his mask loosened onto his chest. He looked my patient in the eye and said,

"John, your daughter got here just in the nick of time. Another hour would have been too late. It was just ready to rupture."

After the doctor left I asked John to get the appendix in a jar and bring it to my office. I wanted to show him the Netter's *Art Collection of Diseased and Normal Structures* to determine whether or not there was anything wrong with her appendix. He brought to my office a healthy little pink appendix preserved in alcohol in a bottle.

'Would have been cancer'

Another statement I hear a lot is, "If I had not removed your tumor, it would have become cancerous."

Fibroid tumors are actually scar tissue, and scar tissue has very poor blood supply. Rarely will you find a malignancy affecting scar tissue.

Gallbladder surgery patients are frequently told that their gallbladders could have ruptured and caused peritonitis.

John, the man whose daughter had the questionable case of appendicitis, came to my office as one of my very first patients and brought his wife in to see me. Their medical doctor wanted to perform a fifth operation in a very short period of time. He advised her to have part of her thyroid gland removed because her basal metabolic rate was a negative 10. I explained to them that a rate between negative 15 and positive 15 is in the normal range.

John was already suspicious because several years earlier, the doctor had advised his wife to have a hysterectomy. John and his wife journeyed to the Mayo Clinic in Rochester, Minnesota, where they found that she did not need a hysterectomy.

After they returned to our local community and advised the doctor of Mayo's findings, the doctor said, "I am not satisfied with their findings. I want her to see a doctor I know in Sioux City, Iowa. He is the best gynecologist in the country."

Sure enough, she needed her uterus removed. The local M.D. persuaded her to have the operation in Sioux City because it would be close to her family, and visitors could come and visit her. This doctor, as stated above, was absolutely the finest in the country.

I found it interesting that by the time John's wife had received the hysterectomy and was back home, the doctor's wife was up at Mayo's having a hysterectomy.

Wouldn't you think that if the Sioux City surgeon was the finest doctor in the country, the doctor would have had his wife's operation performed by him?

Fee splitting and skewing the surgery schedule

When I was interning in a small rural community of Wheatland, Iowa, we had a wonderful old medical country practitioner. When his patients would tell me they had had surgery I would ask them the cost of the operation. They would frequently tell me that the local doctor had given them the check back that the surgeon had sent him for referring the patient.

The practice of sharing the price of a surgical procedure with the referring physician is called fee splitting. The American Academy of Family Physicians is categorically opposed to fee splitting, but trying to stop the practice just made the doctors a little smarter. Technically, fee splitting occurs when no service other than a referral has been provided. Iowa had the reputation as the worst state in the nation for fee splitting. Rather than splitting fees, the referring doctor would "assist" the surgeon in the surgical procedure and therefore collect half the fee.

It was not unusual for the doctors in my area to assist in surgeries performed in a major metropolitan area where three hundred doctors were practicing. There was no need for them to drive sixty-five miles to assist in the surgery they were not capable of doing themselves. Since they were making the trip anyway, it was the custom of many doctors to schedule a number of patients for surgery on the same day and therefore reap the benefit of several surgical assisting fees.

Annabelle, one of my favorite patients from a northwest Iowa community, told me the experience of one of her friends.

The doctor's receptionist called her. "You need to go to the hospital on Sunday evening," she said. "We're going to remove your gallbladder on Monday morning."

She was upset because she had not had any gallbladder problems for more than a year. The receptionist was persistent.

Finally she asked, "What is going on here? Why are you doing this?"

"Oh," the receptionist said, "the doctor had three patients scheduled for surgery. One cancelled, so he wanted to fill the slot."

What some doctors say to encourage patient compliance

The following statements are frequently made by doctors and other care givers in order to put the patient in a fully compliant frame of mind.

- Your appendix was just ready to rupture.
- Another hour would have been too late.
- Without this operation your condition would become cancerous.
- This drug has no side effects.
- This drug has very few side effects.
- This won't hurt.
- During or after your stress test, You need to have this bypass surgery, stent, etc. immediately.
- You could have a heart attack any minute.
- You're sitting on a time bomb.
- If we don't remove your gall bladder it may rupture.
- You're living on borrowed time.
- Are your affairs in order?
- You'd better get your affairs in order!
- Who is your next of kin?
- Stay away from chiropractors. They might injure you. (They have the lowest malpractice rates of any of the healing arts).

- If you were my mother I would advise the same treatment. (Find out if his mother is still living).
- We saved your life. (If the patient dies God called him home).
- Without this procedure you won't last sixty days.

Why you should stay out of hospitals

Many city and regional hospitals today are big business and use the same advertising techniques that other big businesses do. You can see hospital advertising on the sides of buses, on billboards, in the Sunday and weekday newspapers, and during the most popular television programs. They use direct mail, elaborate Web sites, membership programs, and full-color magazines and newsletters to anchor themselves in the minds of the public. They co-sponsor major community events, are active in the local chamber of commerce, and arrange to get their experts interviewed on television and radio talk shows and in meetings of local business organizations.

The most profitable service a hospital can offer is surgery. In California the average cost for major heart surgery is $113,671, but in some hospitals in the state the going rate for the same surgery is $229,962.

Every year more than 72 million surgeries are performed in the United States, forty million of them on an inpatient basis. That comes to one surgical procedure for every four persons or, if you prefer gambling language, you have a one in four chance of undergoing surgery within the next twelve months. And the next year after that. And the next.

One problem with surgery as practiced in this country is that too many of them are ordered and carried out. Before his death Dr. Charles Mayo stated that ninety percent of all surgeries were unnecessary. Back surgeries, according to a 1994 government study, help only one person out of one hundred. Many orthopedic surgeries fail to help the patient. The surgery often ends the athletic career of the person.

Hospitals are the only institute where doctors are furnished technical equipment, nursing staff, continued education and insurance without investing a dime. No other profession is afforded this luxury.

Although, hospitals are necessary under certain conditions, I do my best to avoid going there for myself, my family and my patients. What it costs you to spend a few nights in the hospital you could afford the finest week in Hawaii at a luxury resort. Dr. Mendelson describes a hospital as a place you go to get sick or to die.

Children are especially afraid of hospitals for good reason. There are super germs in hospitals that are resistant to antibiotics. There is understaffing of nursing personnel and frequent mix-ups in drug therapy regimes. You are exposed to all the other illnesses from the patients who share your facilities. A hospital is the temporary repository of animal and vegetable waste from food preparation, biological and diagnostic waste, surgically excised organs, bandages that are soaked with pus, blood and other human excreta, research animals, diapers, catheters, contaminated syringes and fecal material.

You have to remember that the hospital heating and air conditioning system is likely to blow dirt and germs throughout the hospital. Doctors fail to wash their hands unless it is before surgery. They go from room to room palpating and examining sick patients, often without washing their hands between visits.

Even though the customary attire of the hospital personnel is white, there is no way to guarantee the uniforms are free of germs. The soiled bedsheets and operating room drapes, towels, and blankets are all laundered together. How often do you think the hospital sterilizes the mattresses and pillows?

It has been recently reported that 90,000 patients die from exposure to hospitals each year and that two million develop infections from their hospital experience.

Hospitals like to set up rules for keeping visitors away. However, it is the staff that is more likely to contaminate the patients by rotating from ward to ward, room to room and from the lab to the patient's bedside.

We must also consider the drugs that are used in the hospital. Each patient receives an average of 12 different drugs with thousands of possibilities for dangerous interactions. Another danger in the hospital is over exposure to X-rays by CAT scans and X-rays. It is not uncommon for a patient to bring a package of forty X-rays to our clinics with several views of the same structures.

Mistakes made by hospital staff would scare the bravest combat soldier. Surgeons remove the wrong kidney, the wrong arm or the wrong leg. Occasionally babies are mixed up. A classic case happened in Iowa several years ago. The mother sat by who she thought was her badly mangled daughter in the hospital for two weeks and came to find out her daughter had died, and this was some else's daughter. Footprints are not as reliable as fingerprints, and arm bands may fall off.

At the extreme is the fact that doctors and nurses have killed people with injections on purpose. An example was the doctor from England who was responsible for 400 deaths. Recently there was a story on television about a male nurse who injected several people with harmful substances causing their death.

> Malnutrition is one of the most common causes of death in old people in the hospital.

A Boston study concerning nutrition in both American and British hospitals showed that malnutrition is one of the most common causes of death in old people in the hospital because of many disbeliefs of many doctors in vitamins and minerals. The menus are not providing balanced nutrition.

Many times the malnutrition is caused by the patients' refusal to eat because of their drugged state or the stress of their surgeries. Drug therapy frequently robs a person of his or her appetite. Also the patient is ordered not to eat before lab tests. The combination of these facts plus bad food is enough to make anyone malnourished.

It is a matter of public record that many normal appendices are surgically removed all too often. Studies based on autopsy findings show that the diagnosis is wrong fifty percent of the time at our finest medical centers.

You may not realize this, but the hospital can make you sick. Ten percent of all patients hospitalized wind up with infections acquired in the hospital.

American doctors are quick to operate instead of working to prevent disease or treat the patient conservatively. American women, for example, are subjected to five times as many hysterectomies as European women.

Dr. Joel Wallach, author of *Dead Doctors Don't Lie,* did a survey of obituaries in local newspapers and found the average medical doctor died at age fifty-eight. We both believe the reason is taking too many of the drugs that they prescribe to their patients. He also discussed the possibility of 300,000 patients dying each year from medical mishaps from drugs, surgeries and diagnostic procedures.

He stated that forty percent of all hospitalizations are caused by doctors, medicine reactions, and various treatments and examinations.

After losing his wife in 1978 to chemotherapy, Dr. Wallach decided to give up his veterinary practice and went to Naturopathic College and learned to treat patients without drugs and surgery. He has written many books and peer-reviewed articles. He lectures more than three hundred times each year telling patients how to take charge of their health care needs, to avoid doctors, drugs, and surgery whenever possible.

Dr. Wallach believes that the AMA, the FDA, and pharmaceutical companies comprise the Bermuda triangle of health care, the cause of unnumbered medical disasters. He also observed that professional athletes die very young and attributes this to their sweating out the important vitamins and minerals. I believe it's due to the constant physical abuse of their bodies due to the tremendous trauma from sport injuries.

Watch out for sharp objects held by a surgeon

Don't underestimate the might of the surgeon's knife. Rightly applied, it can relieve pain and diseased tissue. In the hands of the overworked or careless physician, surgery can be a terrible mistake.

America leads the world in back surgeries. Our rate of back surgeries per 1,000 population is 500 percent higher than any other developed country.

A government report in 1994 reported that only one patient in 100 was helped by back surgery. A study in *Spine Magazine,* September 2004 illustrated that patients that had back surgery had poorer health status than those patients that did not have back surgery. They scored significantly poorly in all ten scores of the SF-36 Health Survey. A Duke University medical professor reported several years ago that only fifteen percent of all medical procedures proved to be effective.

Almost daily we read about surgeons removing the wrong kidney, the wrong foot, or the wrong lung. Surgeons are removing gall bladders because there happens to be a stone present. Small stones will pass and large stones can't get out. The only time a gall bladder should be removed is when it causes problems.

One of the most popular operations in America is for carpal tunnel syndrome. The February 1994 issue of the *Physical Therapy* reported that only eleven percent of the patients who had that surgery were able to return to their former jobs. Carpal tunnel syndrome can usually be corrected in a chiropractor's office for less than $1,000. Workers' compensation for patients that have surgery for this condition usually runs more than $30,000.

Do you have carpal tunnel syndrome?

Take this simple test. Have someone try to pull a dollar bill from between your thumb and little finger. If you can't hang onto it you may have a carpal tunnel problem. The Hagen clinics have successfully treated hundreds of patients with carpal tunnel problems without surgery.

Too many fatal errors in hospitals

An excellent article entitled "Fixing Hospitals" appeared in the June 20, 2005 issue of *Forbes Magazine*. According to this article 100,000 Americans die every year from medical errors.

That is an understatement. Unfortunately, there are far more fatalities than 100,000. Read or boot up *Death by Medicine* through Google or Yahoo and learn the more accurate figures. Not counting the consequences of other mistakes, ninety thousand patients die of infections acquired in hospital stays each year.

The article states that sixty-one percent of doctors wash their hands before examining a patient if someone is watching. The percentage lowers to forty-one percent if the doctors think no one is watching. I've read reports about cameras that were placed in doctors' lounges, and only twenty-seven percent wash their hands.

During the nineteenth century doctors took over childbirth from midwives, and the mortality rate of infants and mothers rose sharply. Dr. Ignaz Semmelweis observed that doctors went directly from their autopsy labs into crowded maternity wards without washing their hands or changing their clothes. He was sure there was a connection between the substances in the autopsy rooms and the infections of the hospital's patients.

Were his ideas readily accepted? Not at all. The doctor was hounded out of the medical profession and committed to an asylum for the insane. Eventually doctors adopted his suggestions, and infant and maternal death rates dropped significantly.

As it is with all great strides in the healing arts, the majority of doctors reject the new ideas for long periods of time.

In my professional opinion most hospital stays are unnecessary and should be avoided when ever possible. Dr. Robert Mendelson, the author of *Confessions of a Medical Heretic* apparently agrees with my opinion.

He tells about his assignment of twenty-four beds at a Midwestern hospital. When he started weaning out the unnecessary hospital stays and got down to only four patients, they rewarded him by firing him from their staff.

America has almost six thousand hospitals. Wouldn't it be nice to close some of them down? Why do hospitals in the same communities have duplicate services? I recognize that they could both have obstetrical wards but does a community need more than one transplantation hospital? Couldn't two hospitals be operated by the same administrator and eliminate some of those $300,000 salaries?

A casualty count in the *Forbes* article including the following statistics:

- Twenty four percent of people say their family members have been harmed by medical errors. (I think it's much higher. Ask your friends about their experiences.)

- Ninety thousand people succumb to hospital infection.

- One hundred eighty thousand elderly patients die or are seriously injured by drug toxicity.

- Each year seven thousand patients die from drug errors.

- Five hundred fifty-four errors over four months were found at one six-bed intensive care unit; 147 were potentially serious or life-threatening.

- Fifty-five percent of recommended care actually gets administered.

- Employers spend two thousand dollars a year for each insured worker, due to poor-quality care.

- The average wait in an emergency room at a hospital is almost one hour.

I escorted an elderly patient to the emergency room in California three years ago. The patient had tried to swallow a pill that lodged in her throat. She had great difficulty in breathing. The Heimlich maneuver, drinking water, and eating bread failed to dislodge the pill. She waited over an hour before a doctor or nurse saw her.

If a patient's heart stops in an emergency room they only have a fifteen percent chance of surviving.

Mix-ups occur frequently in hospitals. The wrong leg is removed; the wrong knee operated on, the wrong drug or excessive dose is prescribed. The wrong food is served for patients with special dietary needs. Drugs are given that are contraindicated for certain diseases or in combinations with other drugs.

Sometimes babies are mixed up because footprints are not reliable for identifying babies. One hospital in Pennsylvania mixed up their oxygen and nitrous oxide labels. Forty-one deaths occurred before they found their error. My daughter-in-law went into the hospital years ago to have carpal tunnel surgery. After receiving a general anesthetic they started to paint her knees.

An article appeared in the national press last week about a mix-up in hospital supplies where hydraulic fluid was inadvertently used to wash surgical instruments instead of antibacterial soap. The following warning appears in my John Deere Tractor Manual: "Escaping hydraulic fluid may penetrate the skin and cause gangrene. If an accident occurs see a doctor immediately for surgical remove of the fluid."

The *Forbes* article suggests several remedies to lessen the iatrogenesis that occurs in hospitalization. But the best remedy is to take good care of yourself and try to stay out of hospitals.

Our ancestors seldom make us sick

Patients tell me on a daily basis that their condition or illness is genetic. I find this is rarely true.

It is very common for disease to run in families, but not for genetic reasons. If you follow the same lousy diet as your parents did and eat too much sugar, salt, and red meat, if you drink a lot of sodas, are negative in your thinking and live in poor hygienic conditions like those of your parents, you are very likely to develop the same diseases as they did.

A mother that has diabetes and takes insulin during her pregnancy may have a child with Type I diabetes, not because of inheritance but because the insulin she took put her offspring's pancreas to sleep.

Nathan Pritikin stated that if he could change a person's blood chemistries by diet and exercise then their disease wasn't passed on by their genes.

If they ate the same high cholesterol foods as their parents and siblings did, they were going to wind up with high blood pressure, cardiovascular problems, cancer and strokes.

Many diseases run in families, not because they are genetic but because the incidence of certain diseases such as headaches is very high in the general population.

So don't blame it on your genes. Try to find the true cause of your illness.

By the way, you need to be aware of blood transfusions. Maybe the Jehovah Witnesses are right, after all. We now know that blood transfusions increase the mortality risk of heart patients. An increased mortality of 300 percent occurred in 24,000 heart patients receiving blood transfusions within the first thirty days of the transfusions. (*JAMA,* October 6, 2004)

Common medical myths I've heard

I'm amused by the number of half truths and statements of misinformation that people accept as the truth. I'm *not* amused by the consequences of believing myths that have no basis in fact. Disease, suffering, and death can result when you don't pay attention to reality. Here are some common myths I've heard about.

Myth: This drug has no side effects.

Fact: All drugs have multiple and sometimes life-threatening side effects. Between 200,000 and 300,000 people die each year from medically prescribed drugs, according to news reports of recent medical studies.

Myth: You don't need vitamins and minerals. You get all you need in your diet.

Fact: Dr. Emanuel Cheraskin surveyed the eating habits of 15,000 people several years ago. He found that 85 percent of all those surveyed were deficient in at least one nutrient. More than fifty percent were deficient in several vitamins and minerals.

Myth: Going to a chiropractor is dangerous.

Fact: Chiropractors have the lowest malpractice rates of any of the healing arts, a strong testimony of the safety of their practices.

Myth: There's no such thing as a pinched nerve. Fifty years ago the medical profession claimed that chiropractors couldn't help a patient because a vertebrae couldn't get out of alignment far enough to pinch a nerve.

Fact: Guess what? MRIs, CAT Scans, and EMGs have all proven the possibility of nerves being pinched. Chiropractors were right all along.

Myth: If a medical doctor tells you a chiropractor can't help you for a certain condition, find a new doctor.

Fact: Only a chiropractor knows whether or not you are a chiropractic case.

Myth: Chiropractors are not well trained.

Fact: As long as fifty years ago chiropractors were required to pass the same examination in most states that the medical doctors and osteopaths took. Tests chiropractors take include tests in anatomy, physiology, chemistry, bacteriology, pathology, and hygiene and sanitation. I know of twenty-five medical doctors studying chiropractic today that would attest to the quality of chiropractic education.

Myth: Chiropractors can only help back and neck problems.

Fact: Every cell, tissue, organ, or system in your body is controlled directly or indirectly by your nervous system. All nerves, with the exception of the twelve cranial nerves, must pass through the vertebrae in the spine in order to control all body functions. Spinal misalignments or subluxations can cause many diseases.

Myth: Chiropractors claim they can cure everything by spinal manipulation.

Fact: Chiropractors don't claim to cure anything. As far as they're concerned, only hams are cured. Chiropractors correct subluxations or spinal misalignments, restoring a normal or better nerve supply to the sick cells, tissues, organs, or systems—and the body cures itself. A medical doctor doesn't heal a broken arm. He merely puts the ends together. The miracle of healing is produced by your body's inborn intelligence.

Myth: Medical doctors are well trained in the subject of nutrition.

Fact: Most medical doctors receive very little training in the science of nutrition.

Myth: Medical science is curing a lot of cancers nowadays.

Fact: Cancer kills three times as many people today as it did fifty years ago. The most feared diagnosis in medicine today is "cancer." Fortunately, some people survive in spite of treatment by surgery, radiation, and chemotherapy. One of the most successful treatments of cancer came from strengthening the patient's immune system by vitamin therapy, biofeedback, hugging, and prayers—as reported by the Harvard School of Medicine. Fortunately, eighty to ninety percent of all cancers can be prevented by avoiding smoking and drinking, eating fruits and vegetables, breathing clean air and drinking pure water, avoiding toxic chemicals and overcooked fatty meats, exercising, taking vitamins and certain minerals, reducing fatty foods, and eating whole grain foods. Why hasn't modern medicine addressed prevention rather than treating the cancers by expensive therapies of questionable value?

Myth: New medical developments result in the curing of a lot of diseases other than cancer.

Fact: Name one disease that medicine can cure today. Not arthritis, diabetes, AIDS, influenza, the common cold, migraine, heart disease, high blood pressure, MS, cancer, fibromyalgia, psoriasis, and on and on. Most medicines either stimulate or inhibit function. They do not normalize function.

Myth: Americans live a lot longer today than they did a century ago.

Fact: According to the three medical specialists and a CEO who wrote the book, *Sugar Busters*, an American who is fifty years old today will live only eighteen months longer than a person who was fifty years old in 1900. The biggest difference in longevity tables is due to a reduction in infant mortality. Heart attacks, lung cancer, strokes, and diabetes were rare in 1900.

Myth: Americans are healthier than people in any other nation.

Fact: In America our life expectancy at birth of 77.4 puts us behind other 28 countries. We also have the highest infant mortality rate among the eleven most affluent countries.

Myth: Back surgery will cure slipped, ruptured, or herniated discs.

Fact: Back surgery is successful only one percent of the time, according to a 1994 government study by twenty-seven specialists.

Myth: Carpal tunnel surgery will restore people to the work force.

Fact: According to the *Physical Therapy Journal* (February, 1994), eighty-nine percent of patients having carpal tunnel surgery were unable to perform or return to their former job. Carpal tunnel injuries have become one of America's most expensive workers' compensation problems. Most carpal tunnel problems are caused by a pinched nerve in the neck, leading to the muscles and ligaments in the hand.

Myth: All medical procedures are based on scientific studies and research.

Fact: An Associated Press report on January 12, 2000, reported that the Federal Trade Commission had charged that a series of Bayer ads made unsubstantiated claims that regular aspirin use could help the general public prevent heart attacks and strokes. The report stated that there's little evidence that aspirin prevents a heart attack in someone who doesn't already have vascular disease, said Dr. Rodman Starke of the American Heart Association. The side effects of aspirin can harm some people.

Myth: Americans have one of the best diets in the world.

Fact: Americans eat too much meat, drink too many soft drinks (they should be called "hard" drinks because they're hard on your health), eat too much sugar, white flour, and white rice; too much fat and too little fiber (that's why we're so constipated), and too much ice cream. Two thirds of adult males half of adult females are obese; one quarter of our children are significantly overweight. Is this because we have the best diet in the world? Hardly. Our breakfast cereals are more sugar than substance. A ten-ounce can of pop may contain ten teaspoons of sugar. Would you let your child dump ten teaspoons of sugar on the breakfast food? Most youngsters today drink more sodas than water. With all that sugar and fat in their diet, is it any wonder they have to be treated for acne? If you could package cholesterol in a box, I'm sure there would be a ready market for it in the U.S.

Myth: We need more salt in our diet.

Fact: Americans consume ten to twenty times as much salt as they need in their diet. While sodium chloride is essential for many body functions, excess salt may raise your blood pressure, damage your kidneys, and cause swelling of the ankles. Salt is ubiquitous. It is packaged in almost everything we eat or drink. I haven't used a salt shaker in the past twenty years, but every time I have a blood test I show high levels of sodium and chloride.

Myth: I don't need chiropractic care.

Fact: If you have a spine you need a chiropractor to keep it properly aligned. If you have teeth, you need a dentist. If you have eyes you need an eye doctor. If you have feet you need a podiatrist, especially when you get older. If your nerves lead from your brain, down your spine to the organs and tissues of your body, doesn't it make sense to keep your spine lined up?

When to call a physician

Most doctors would be honest enough to tell you that the majority of visits to doctors' offices are unnecessary and not productive. However, there are times when medical visits are imperative. Listed below is a list of signs and symptoms that merit visits without delay:

- Severe trauma
- Fainting, dizziness, or unconsciousness
- Double vision or loss of vision
- High body temperature
- Shortness of breath
- Choking
- Irregular heart beat
- Blood in the urine
- Blood in the stool, especially tar colored stools

- Excessive loss or gain in weight
- Loss of speech and inability to whistle
- Severe pain in the chest, over the heart, throat, or down the left arm
- Swelling of lymph glands in neck, armpits, or groin
- Swelling of the ankles with pitting or elastic sock marks
- High blood pressure
- Sores or wounds that don't heal quickly
- Severe numbness and weakness of the arms and legs
- Severe pain under the right side of the rib cage and under the right shoulder blade
- Severe pain in the lower right quadrant of the abdomen
- Excessive thirst
- Incoherence
- Suspected drug reactions
- Chronic coughing
- Urinary or bowel incontinence or inability to move bowels or pass urine

Watch out for medications

If we threw all the medicine in the
world into the sea it would be so much
the better for mankind and so much
the worse for the fish.

—Dr. Oliver Wendell Holmes
Former president, Harvard Medical School

Drug companies distribute over 5,000 news releases weekly to newspapers and magazines touting the benefits of new drugs. Every year 1,500 new drugs come into the marketplace. Every year many drugs are removed from the market because of potential adverse side effects.

Researchers who are paid to skew their reports in favor of the sponsoring drug company compromise research of new drugs. Up to 95 percent of drug research is associated with doctors paid by the various drug companies.

The Food and Drug Administration is suspect for protecting the drug companies more than they are protecting the public. They are notorious for going after vitamin companies and ignoring deaths cause by various drugs.

Many times the drug companies hire the former Food and Drug Administration director to expedite the approval process for drugs that should have never entered the market in the first place.

A Duke University medical expert recently stated that eighty-five percent of all medical procedures were not scientifically proven by double-blind studies.

Some doctors seem to believe that every patient that leaves his or her office needs to have a new prescription in hand. The side effects of three or four different drugs are absolutely unpredictable.

Pharmaceutical companies constantly place ads in magazines touting the wonderful benefits of their drugs. If you read the fine print on the back page of the drug ads, you would be concerned about the side effects that you may encounter. To quote Dr. Thomas Pluess, "There is not a cure in a carload of medicine."

Even Sioux Falls has a serious drug problem. I'm not talking about drugs sold in dark alleys. I'm talking about prescribed and over-the-counter drugs. It's not unusual for patients visiting our office to be taking as many as fifty pills a day. God only knows the terrible side effects that could and does occur from drug combinations.

The Journal of the American Medical Association reported that legally prescribed drugs cause more than 100,000 deaths each year. That makes it the fourth leading cause of death following heart attacks, strokes, and diabetes.

Twenty percent of all dialysis patients are taking this treatment because they took over-the-counter drugs such as Nuprin, Motrin, Aleve, Advil, and Naproxen, according to the *Los Angeles Times.*

Near the end of 2004, *MD Medical News* reported that Aleve, a popular pain-killing drug, has been added to the list of NSAIDs linked to heart attacks.

The National Institutes of Health suspended a large Alzheimer's prevention trial after it discovered that healthy elderly patients taking Aleve increased their risk of strokes and heart attacks by fifty percent.

There is no need to indict specific brand names of dangerous drugs. As FDA Commissioner Dr. Lester Crawford said when he appeared on the Today Show, any drug taken at high dosages for a prolonged period of time can cause serious problems.

Twenty-five hundred healthy elderly people were involved in a three-year program designed to see if Aleve or Celebrex prevented Alzheimer's disease.

Those in the experiment had a fifty percent increased risk of stroke or heart attack compared to those who received a placebo in the double blind study.

Dr. John Breitner, MD, MPH, head researcher, stated that no evidence of other NSAIDs supported the idea that they were any safer in terms of heart attack risk.

The respected medical journal, *The Lancet,* included a report in its October 2, 2004, edition suggesting that steroid treatment for head injuries may cause death. The study reported that 10,000 patients treated with head injuries were more likely to die in a two-week period if they had been treated with corticosteroids. A seventeen percent greater mortality rate occurred in the steroid users.

Other medical studies found that the arthritis drug Remicade increases the risk of lymphoma threefold, increased susceptibility to tuberculosis and a lowering of white blood cells and platelets has been observed. The drug is frequently prescribed for rheumatoid arthritis patients.

NSAID is the abbreviation for a family of medicines taken by millions of people every day to decrease fever, swelling, and redness. The medical name is "nonsteroidal anti-inflammatory drug."

> NSAIDs such as aspirin, Anacin, Bufferin, Excedrin and the ibuprofen drugs such as Aleve, Nuprin, Motrin, Advil, and Naproxen can cause injury to the small intestines.

A medical study reported in 2004 found that frequent and continued use of NSAIDs such as aspirin, Anacin, Bufferin, Excedrin and the ibuprofen drugs such as Aleve, Nuprin, Motrin, Advil, and Naproxen cause injury to the small intestines. Seventy-one percent of the frequent users had inflammation of the small intestine, small erosions, or large erosions and ulcers. Sixteen thousand deaths occur each year from using NSAIDs. That's almost as many people as those that die from AIDS.

According to an article in the January 12, 2000 *The Desert Sun* (Palm Springs, California), the Bayer Company, according to the Federal Trade Commission, made unsubstantiated claims that regular aspirin use could help prevent heart attacks and strokes.

Dr. Rodman Starke of the American Heart Association stated there is little evidence that aspirin prevents heart attack in someone who doesn't already have vascular disease. Aspirin also has deleterious side effects.

Another aspirin study
The 20,000 participants in the 10-year Women's Health Study who took 100 milligrams of aspirin every other day were no less likely to suffer heart attacks than did women in the study who took placebos.

Several years ago 22,000 U.S. doctors were given a daily aspirin to see if the daily use of aspirin would prevent heart attacks, and the study did find that aspirin was effective in preventing heart attacks. The same study was conducted in England and reported in the *British Medical Journal* with the additional comment that aspirin increased the risk of strokes.

Ironically, the study was sponsored and financed by the Bayer Company. One should always question the validity of any study with the potential of benefiting the sponsor.

The prescription arthritis drug Vioxx has recently been reported as increasing your chance of heart failure by eighty percent.

Elderly people living in Ontario, Canada, were divided into groups taking Vioxx, Celebrex, ibuprofen products, and one that took no drugs. For the ibuprofen group, the risk of heart failure increased by forty percent. Ibuprofen products also increased the risk of kidney failure.

While increased risk was not present among Celebrex takers, the results were similar to the those of the participants who took no drugs.

Approximately one in four Americans has arthritis or other diseases of their joints. I recommend arthritis sufferers to find a good chiropractor, a massage therapist, and a nutritionist. Dietary changes should include eliminating sugar, eating as organically as possible and taking fish liver oils.

Are pills ever necessary? Of course. My wife had eye surgery to correct her vision so she could read without glasses. Because of the irritation of the surgery, she had a prescription lotion applied to her eye. Other than that, my wife has gone her entire life without taking a prescription.

Popping drugs by the handful

Forbes Magazine dated November 29, 2004, included an article by Robert Langreth entitled "Pharma's New Enemy: Clean Living." The author questions the need for all the prescription drugs that Americans are popping by the handful. He points out that we are popping dangerous drugs for innocuous ills that could be prevented and cured by diet, exercise, and clean living—a far less expensive and dangerous approach to good health.

Langreth's estimate of two million complications and 180,000 deaths caused by prescription drugs is much more conservative than Gary Nulls' book, *Death by Medicine* which researched iatrogenesis reported by all the specialties and came up with 768,000 deaths per year caused by doctors and prescribed drugs.

A good example is the recent Vioxx scandal, a drug produced by Merck. Patients injured and dying are reported to number 30,000 to 100,000. We are already seeing lawyer ads in newspapers and on television seeking clients wishing to sue Merck.

The general public should realize they don't need to pop a pill for every pain. Drug prescriptions are increasing at the rate of fifteen percent each year. A Harvard Medical School instructor is quoted as saying drug manufacturers are exaggerating the benefits and minimizing the side effects of drugs instead of encouraging clean living.

Dr. Dean Ornish and Nathan Pritikin have long advocated that a plethora of diseases can be cured and prevented by exercise and a diet low in fat, sugar, salt, and refined foods.

Drug interactions to avoid

It seems like doctors are prescribing Prednisone at the drop of a hat. This drug, a synthetic cortisone, comes with a plethora of serious side effects. It may make you feel energetic and wonderful for a time, but its adverse effects may not be worth the temporary gains. It may lead to diabetes, and fractures may occur from the depletion of calcium, Vitamin D, potassium and B vitamins.

Antibiotics like Cipro, Noroxin, and tetracycline should not be taken with calcium-fortified orange juice, milk, cheese, and other dairy products, or calcium supplements because calcium interferes with antibiotic therapy.

Grapefruit and grapefruit juice interfere with the absorption of many drugs, especially blood pressure drugs. Cipro magnifies the effects of caffeine.

Food, vitamins, tea, juice and coffee should not be taken less than one hour before or after taking Fosamax. If you lie down after taking Fosamax it may ulcerate your esophagus.

Estrogen: one of medicine's greatest boondoggles

For more than forty years American women were advised that they needed estrogen to replace their declining natural levels of this important hormone.

Common drugs in this category of medicines, prescribed as HRT (hormone replacement therapy) are Premarin, Provera and Prempro. The public was assured that HRT prevented heart attacks, strokes, breast cancers, Alzheimer's Disease, and osteoporosis.

At its peak, four out of ten women were taking or had taken some form of HRT. It was unusual for postmenopausal women to enter my clinic who weren't taking "HRT." I never permitted my wife to take these medicines and advised as many women as I could to gradually get off estrogen.

A research program known as the Women's Health Initiative was established to measure the effects of combination hormone replacement therapy. The massive program was discontinued in 2002 by the federal government because of the deleterious side effects of HRT.

The results of taking HRT as discovered from evidence revealed in the Women's Health Initiative were published in the *Essential Guide to Prescription Drugs 2004*.

They included the following bad effects of HRT:

1. Increased risk of breast cancer.

2. Increased risk of heart attack.

3. Increased risk of stroke.

4. Increased risk of deep vein clots.

5. Increased risk of cancer of the uterus.

6. Accelerated growth of fibroid tumors.

7. Fluid retention.

8. Postmenopausal bleeding.

9. Increased gall stone risk.

10. Increased high blood pressure risk.

11. Decreased sugar tolerance.

I've also read recently that instead of protecting women from Alzheimer's Disease, HRT doubles the risk.

During 1981 I published what was then the largest nutritional chart ever published. At that time one of my scientific sources for this project stated that estrogen caused osteoporosis. Nevertheless, for many years women were given estrogen to prevent osteoporosis.

What a boondoggle.

> **Dementia drugs**
>
> A 3-month study at the University of Southern California found a fifty percent higher death rate among elderly patients treated for dementia with antipsychotic drugs compared to those on placebos. The study involved 5,000 persons and was reported in *JAMA,* Oct. 19, 2005.

Painkillers can make you worse

Frequent use of painkillers may actually make you sick. A May 11, 2004 study reported in *Neurology* states that the daily use of analgesics may cause chronic headaches, chronic migraines, and, occasionally, neck and back pain.

Sixty thousand patients age twenty or over were surveyed for the study. Chronic headache sufferers were defined as those that experience headaches fifteen days each month. Migraine diagnosis was predicated on those headaches lasting four to seventy-two hours, aggravated by activity, one sided, and pulsating veins.

Daily use of analgesics for one month or more was considered overuse. The findings showed that patients taking analgesics daily for six months were twenty times more likely to suffer chronic migraines. They were also three and one half times more likely to suffer from neck and back pain.

Previous peer review studies have demonstrated that many medicines result in joint and disc damage.

The researchers' conclusions stated, "The high numbers of individuals with analgesic overuse has important clinical implications, and physicians should be aware of the potential risk of analgesic overuse among those with chronic pain, especially those with migraines."

It seems the best treatment for these symptoms would be to get off the drugs.

The FDA and drug makers

The FDA ignored repeated warnings about the contamination of the flu vaccine manufactured by Chiron. Dangerous bacteria were found to cause contamination over a period of five years. Twenty problems were found during a 2003 inspection of Chiron's Liverpool plant, many of them going back to 1999.

Contamination rather than the killed virus in the vaccine is responsible for the occasional violent reactions people experience after a vaccination, such as paralysis and even death.

According to my local newspaper dated December 27, 2004, the FDA issued a belated warning about the use and abuse of NSAID drugs. The use of these over-the-counter drugs such as aspirin, naproxen, Advil, Nuprin, Motrin, Celebrex, Bextra and Aleve for more than ten days is contraindicated without a doctor's supervision. The FDA also advises patients not to take more than the amount of medication recommended on the label.

Dr. David Graham, whistle blower on Merck's Vioxx drug, estimates that 139,000 deaths or serious injuries occurred over the last few years from taking Vioxx. He warns that the FDA is often too quick to approve drugs with serious side effects and has testified against the user of Accutane, for acne; Serevent for asthma; Meridia for weight reduction; and Bextra for arthritis and pain management. All of these drugs have serious issues, he says.

Harvard Medical School professor and author Dr. Jerry Avom says he believes that the FDA takes better care of the drug companies than of the prescription users.

On Wednesday, January 5, 2005, the headline reads, "For those in pain, relief trumps risks of medications." Sub-headline: "Bad news of recent weeks leaves many patients with tough choices."

The painkilling drugs Vioxx Celebrex, Bextra, and Aleve have been blamed by many scientists for causing a plethora of problems for patients taking them.

A 2001 study designed to prove that these four drugs were superior to previous OTC drugs showed that between 88,000 to 139,000 users of Vioxx suffered heart attacks with a thirty percent possibility of fatality.

The National Cancer Society halted two studies involving Vioxx that were expected to show a decrease in colon cancer and risk of Alzheimer's disease. The risk of heart attack from the use of Vioxx doubled.

CNN News, *Lou Dobbs Tonight,* February 28, 2005: The program featured an interview with Dr. John Abramson, author of the book *Overdose America: The Broken Promise of American Medicine.*

Dr. Abramson told the television audience that ten of the thirty-two doctors on the oversight board that recently reversed the withdrawal of Vioxx and put it back on the market had drug company connections. Had these doctors with a vested financial interest in drug companies been disqualified, the vote would have been fourteen to eight preventing Vioxx from future sales.

According to Abramson, Vioxx is a twenty billion dollar per year drug. He also stated that doctors are victims just like patients when it comes to evaluating the efficacy of drugs. They don't have the time from their busy practice schedules to research the drugs they prescribe. Negative reports about Vioxx and other harmful drugs do not reach them, and many doctors are not reading their journals.

The report also stated that drugs companies fund eighty percent of trials. Therefore those trials have a built-in bias favoring the drug companies. You can buy this book from Amazon.com.

Another book available from Amazon is *The Truth About the Drug Companies: How They Deceive Us and What to do About It.* The author is Marcia Angell, former editor-in-chief of the *New England Journal of Medicine.* She states that pharmaceutical companies are fraught with corruption and doing a disservice for patients, the federal government, and the medical establishment itself.

> Most research and development of new drugs is done by colleges and universities and paid for by the government.

Although drug companies claim that it costs 800 million dollars to bring a drug to market she points out a huge portion of that expense goes into marketing rather than research. Most research and development is done by colleges and universities and paid for by the government.

Other books for reading include, *On the Take: How Medical Complicity with Big Business Can Endanger Your Health; Critical Condition: How Health Care in America Became Big Business—and Bad Medicine; Overdose: The Case Against the Drug Companies: Prescription Drugs, Side Effects, and Your Health.*

America leads the world in developing new treatment protocols, drugs, technology and surgeries, but ranks a lowly twenty-ninth in longevity. America also leads the world in marketing drugs with $25 million spent on advertising to doctors which amounts to about $36,000 per doctor. Drug companies aren't satisfied with merely advertising to doctors. Now the general public is bombarded with television, radio, magazine, and newspaper ads extolling the benefits of drugs, but try to hide their potential side effects. You're advised repeatedly to ask your doctor for a prescription for the latest "wonder drug." The doctor has his ethics compromised by acquiescing to your demands.

Drug companies have emphasized the promotion of Lipitor or other statin drugs for healthy people even though half of the heart attack victims have normal cholesterol levels. When I attended college the normal cholesterol levels were up to 250. Now drug companies encourage lower levels because every time they lower the normal levels, ten million more patients fall into the category of spending one hundred dollars per month on a drug with side effects that include severe muscle damage, death, and the reduction of CoQ-10 levels in your body by twenty-five percent. CoQ-10 does prevent heart attacks from occurring.

Another drug with unexpected side effects is the arthritis drug Remicade, which increases the risk of lymphoma threefold. The drug is frequently prescribed for rheumatoid arthritis patients. Susceptibility to tuberculosis also results from the drug, and a lowering of WBCs and platelets has been observed.

Questions surround oversight of the drug industry

A strong majority of FDA scientists feel the agency does a poor job of monitoring drugs.

Two-thirds of Food and Drug Administration professionals are less than fully confident in the agency's monitoring of the safety of prescription drugs now being sold, according to an FDA internal survey. One third are concerned about the process of approving new drugs. This survey was conducted in 2001

Dr. David Graham, who blew the whistle on Vioxx and five other drugs, was praised on national television by Senator Charles Grassley of Iowa, who proposed an oversight committee to investigate and reform the FDA. Grassley has chastised the FDA for failing to protect American citizens from death and serious injuries from the arthritis drug Vioxx and antidepressants that produce suicidal potentials in our American youths.

His comments released to Iowa newspapers during November of 2004 stated that Vioxx may have resulted in 30,000 to 100,000 heart attacks, strokes, and other major iatrogenic reactions among its users. The FDA, according to Grassley, may have tried to sweep under the rug a possible link between anti-depressant drugs and suicidal behavior among adolescents.

Grassley also claims the many suits that are arising from drug injuries will markedly increase the cost of other medicines while consumers are already unhappy about the high costs of drugs.

On December 17, 2004, major TV medical news pointed out that Celebrex research has shown that patients that took that drug were two and a half to three and a half times more likely to suffer a heart attack than nonusers of the drug.

My sister-in-law started bleeding from the bowels after taking Celebrex for knee pain. She had been warned by her doctor son and grandsons not to take it.

I predict that Celebrex may go the way of Vioxx before long.

The FDA and the drug problem

During a recent week the following headline appeared in several publications: "FDA ignored vaccine warning." The report went on to say that the FDA had failed to heed warnings that a British flu vaccine manufacturer was producing contaminated and unsafe vaccines. The FDA left it up to Chiron to correct the problem voluntarily. Actually, the British government and authorities shut down production after they found dangerous bacterial problems with the vaccine.

One news source reported the vaccine had been contaminated since 1999. One thousand pages of documents by the FDA, Chiron, and British health authorities were presented to a congressional hearing. The FDA was made aware of the contamination problems over the past several years, but it was the British regulators that finally closed down the plant. The FDA inspection team found twenty problems in June of 2003, but did nothing to protect the American public from receiving 100 million doses of contaminated vaccine during the fall of 2003.

WebMD reported on November 19, 2004, that Dr. David Graham, an FDA scientist, had accused the FDA of bowing to drug makers. Speaking to the Senate Finance Committee, Dr. Graham testified that the FDA was failing at its job of ensuring safety for patients taking drugs. Graham told lawmakers that the FDA was incapable of protecting Americans from another Vioxx, the widely used drug recently removed from the market by its manufacturer Merck. He also warned that five other prescription drugs should be closely monitored due to safety concerns. These drugs included Crestor, Bextra, Meridia, Serevent, and Accutane.

Graham wisely called for an independent monitoring free of influence from regulators that approve new drugs.

Patients taking any drugs should be aware that there is no such thing as a safe drug. A pharmacist recently told me that her pharmacy professor reminded her class every day that every drug is a poison.

Public Citizen's director, Dr. Sidney Wolfe, has petitioned the FDA to remove Crestor from the market because the cholesterol drug is seventy-five times more likely to cause kidney damage than other statin drugs.

Consumer advocates are reminded that many times serious side effects are not discovered until after a drug has been used for several years.

The FDA approved Mifeprex in 2000 to terminate pregnancy up to 49 days. In the summer of 2005 the FDA issued a black box warning against the abortion pill Mifeprex to highlight safety concerns about its use. The use of RU-486 apparently had been the primary cause of a serious bacterial infection and death of an 18-year-old woman from California the previous year.

Critics of the FDA say the organization acts too quickly in the approval of certain drugs and fails to properly monitor their serious side effects.

Dr. Jerry Avorn, Harvard Medical School professor and renowned author, hit the nail on the head when he stated that the FDA was taking better care of the drug companies than of the prescription users. Dr. Avorn accused the FDA of submitting to pressure from drug companies to get drugs on the market without addressing unresolved safety issues.

The selling of drugs

Drug ads are ubiquitous. They encourage patients to ask their doctors to prescribe drugs advertised in the various media. If the doctor refuses their request, they are urged to find another doctor.

False and misleading ads create demands for unsafe and questionable drugs. The ads extol the virtues of the drug while minimizing the potential deleterious effects.

Drug advertising expenditures have mushroomed 400 percent in the past seven years. An increase of fifteen percent or more prescriptions is taking place annually.

The biggest problem is the co-mingling of many pharmacy products without knowing the adverse effects of those multiple compounds.

Doctors testified at the AMA meeting in Chicago that unproven drugs are getting into the hands of patients who do not need them.

The FDA eased advertising restrictions in 1997. Are we any healthier today as a result? Vioxx was one of the most heavily advertised drugs on the market. After causing thousands of heart attacks and deaths it was removed from the market temporarily. It is now back on the market after a panel of twenty-six doctors approved it. Ten of the panel doctors recommending restoring its sales had investments in drug companies.

There are more drug lobbyists in Washington than there are senators and congressmen. Go figure.

At the end of June the AMA delegates voted not to restrict drug advertising.

Why drugs cost so much

Once the medications are developed, branded, and advertised, there is one more step that pushes the cost still higher.

Branded drugs cost the consumer as much as 2,000 percent more than generic equivalents. Much of this cost increase is due to markups by the final seller of the product, the pharmacy. For example, consumer investigators found that Enalapril, the generic form of Vasotec, a widely prescribed high blood pressure medication, costs pharmacies about $5 for a month's supply. Walgreen charges about $67 for the same prescripton. Famoltidine, the generic equivalent of the well-known acid-reducing medication, Pepcid, costs your pharmacy about $6 but sells for $97 at CVS and $98 at Rite Aid. Your pharmacy pays about $4 for a month's supply of Fluoxetine, the generic equivalent of the anti-depressant drug Prozac. CVS will charge you $79, and Rite Aid's price is $82.

Investigators found that reasonably priced prescription drugs could be found in stores like WalMart and KMart. The best prices were at Costco, where Enalpril sells for $12.08, Famotidine for $12.24, and Fluoxetine for $9.63. Costco company officials say they still make a profit even with their low prices and do not require membership for persons buying prescription drugs.

The use and misuse of antibiotics

The wonder drugs of the twentieth century were the antibiotics. Their development led to drastic reductions in the morbidity and mortality of mankind and livestock from infectious diseases. Unfortunately, because of their excessive use and abuse by physicians and the prescribing of antibiotics for viral conditions, many disease organisms are now resistant to treatment.

Antibiotics are only effective in treating bacterial diseases. They do not destroy viruses. Viruses cause the common cold, flu, chickenpox, measles, mumps and many other diseases.

There are over 2,000 bacteria. Only about one hundred are harmful to mankind. The E-coli in your intestinal tract are necessary for the absorption and putrefaction that takes place in your intestinal track. Most antibiotics kill bacteria regardless of whether or not they are beneficial or pathological.

Therefore, when you take antibiotics you destroy the good as well as the harmful germs. When you destroy the E-coli in your body you become more susceptible to yeast infections. I always advise anyone taking antibiotics to take lactobacillus acidophilus to replace the natural flora of their intestinal track.

> Antibiotics destroy good as well as bad germs. When you destroy the E-coli in your body you become more susceptible to yeast infections.

Staphylococcus aureus, the organism that is the major cause of hospital infections, has developed a resistance to antibiotics in the penicillin class as well as to the macrolides.

The best way to avoid antibiotic therapy is to avoid getting infections. A good vitamin regime, especially the ingestion of vitamins A and C, and the minerals zinc and selenium, fresh air, natural sunlight, physical exercise, sufficient rest, washing your hands, and avoiding stress will do much to maintain a high level of immunity. I've not missed a day of work in over fifty-five years due to illness.

Before taking an antibiotic, make certain a proper diagnosis of a bacterial infection has been made. Many articles have been published in peer reviewed journals lately about the overuse of antibiotics in treating ear infections in children.

An article in the *Los Angeles Times* several years ago told about a football player who took Advil for a sprained ankle. This commonly used over-the-counter drug ruined his kidneys and ended his professional football career. The article went on to say that twenty percent of all dialysis patients ended up on dialysis after taking ibuprofen products such as Advil, Motrin, Aleve, and Nuprin.

There has been a three hundred percent increase in kidney failures since these potentially dangerous drugs have been sold without a prescription. Yet many doctors continue to recommend high dosages for their patients.

At the Hagen Clinic patients on these drugs show albumin and blood in their urine when a urinalysis is performed. These two abnormal constituents of urine reveal that the kidneys are being damaged.

Sir Alexander Fleming, discoverer of penicillin, visited the United States during the fifties. While here he had a cold. He visited a doctor for his cold and reported to the press that normally it took a week to get over a cold in England but in America it took him a week to get over his cold, a week to get over the drug the doctor prescribed for him and a third week to get over the doctor bill.

During the fifties it was customary for doctors to give penicillin regardless of the diagnosis. If the patient didn't get well in a week they would then exam the patient. I remember one patient told me he visited his family doctor with pain in his shoulder and was given a shot of penicillin. No wonder we have millions of people allergic to penicillin.

Colds, influenza, and most childhood diseases are viral diseases. Several articles have appeared in the national news of late concerning the over prescribing of antibiotics for ear infections.

Remember that antibiotics are only effective against bacterial infections. If you're suffering from a viral infection, antibiotics will do you more harm than good.

Side effects of antibiotics

The following possible side effects of the use of antibiotics are listed in *The Merck Manual of Medical Information, Home Edition*:

Hearing loss; vertigo; kidney damage; diarrhea; gastrointestinal upset, nausea and vomiting; allergic reaction, anaphylactic shock (may result in death); brain, liver, and kidney damage; nerve damage; skin rashes; kidney failure; decreased white blood cell count; sensitivity to sunlight; discoloration of the teeth, potential toxicity to mother and fetus if used during pregnancy, eye damage; seizures, and low blood pressure; metallic taste; dark urine and increased uric acid levels; hepatitis; red-orange saliva, tears, sweat, and urine; fever and chills; confusion, seizures, and coma; nervousness, toxic reaction to bone marrow; anemia and clotting problems, inflammation of the pancreas and of the eyes and eyelids when applied to the eyes; kidney stones; fatigue; flu-like symptoms; headaches; hair loss; breakdown of red blood cells; stinging of the eyes; lowered blood potassium levels; inner ear damage; and blocked production of testosterone and cortisol.

A doctor must weigh the seriousness of the infection against the risk of antibiotic reactions. Many of the toxic side effects are unpredictable. It is important to avoid the use and abuse of antibiotics whenever possible because overuse of these drugs has caused many disease organisms to become resistant to antibiotics.

Aspirin can be dangerous

Aspirin may cause internal bleeding and Reye's Syndrome in children who receive aspirin for the flu or chickenpox. Reye's Syndrome is usually fatal.

Aspirin robs your body of folic acid, and pregnant women with folic acid deficiencies may have a baby with a cleft palate or spina bifida. Aspirin consumption also may cause a deficiency of vitamin K, B_1, B_{12}, and C.

The Bayer Company was fined a million dollars years ago by the Federal Trade Commission for claiming that regular use of aspirin would prevent heart attacks and strokes.

People should think twice before taking two aspirin.

The Mayo Clinic conducted a Liver Transplantation Seminar in Minneapolis at the Sofitel Hotel during the fall of 1999. Doctors attending that seminar were told that seventy thousand liver failures occur annually worldwide. Thirty-five thousand occur from AIDS and diabetes and the remaining thirty-five thousand are from taking Tylenol and other over-the-counter drugs. Tylenol is especially harmful taken with alcohol or anticonvulsant drugs. Liver failures are life-threatening because the liver performs up to five hundred functions for your welfare.

The fewer drugs, the better

After over fifty years of practice I find it rare to have to use drugs to help a patient recover from an illness. I went fifty years without using an aspirin, Tylenol, or ibuprofen product. My wife has never had a prescription drug in our first fifty-three years of marriage.

Most maladies have remedies that do not require medicine to alleviate their symptoms. Most medicines only cover up symptoms. They do not correct the cause of disease. The one thing I like about the Mayo Clinic is they usually take away more drugs than they prescribe.

One of my favorite medical doctors in Sioux Falls is board certified in eight medical specialties and is one of the smartest men I've ever known. He does everything he can to avoid giving drugs to patients.

I bought a book last year entitled *The Essential Guide to Prescription Drugs 2004* co-authored by James J. Ryback, a doctor of pharmacy. The subtitle reads, "Everything you need to know for safe drug use."

If you read the description of the side effects of the drugs you're taking, you'll probably throw them away. For instance, one of the side effects of aspirin is hemorrhagic stroke.

If you are taking two or more drugs at the same time it's almost unpredictable what the side effects might be. Remember every drug is a poison and that ibuprofen products cause kidney failure. Acetaminophen (Tylenol) causes 35,000 liver failures each year according to the Mayo Clinic.

There's no such thing as a safe drug.

Do everything you can to avoid taking drugs. Chiropractic, massage therapy, vitamins, acupuncture, and physical therapy are good alternatives to drugs and surgery.

Prescription drugs

Whenever a doctor prescribes a drug to a non-pregnant patient that patient ought to ask the doctor the following questions:

1. What is the mechanism of action of this drug?

2. What are the side effects of this drug? Ask for a full description and *read it.*

3. Can this medicine react with my other medications?

4. Can I get a generic, less expensive form of that drug?

5. How soon can I quit taking the drug?

Getting free samples of drugs from your doctor is not always a good thing. Many times doctors are paid to give out free samples and then to report the efficacy or toxic side effects of a particular drug. If the doctor does not write a good report for the drug he no longer gets paid or receives free samples.

Doctors are also known to over prescribe drugs that they have a stock investment in.

Forty years ago I told a schoolteacher friend of mine how surprised I was to learn that my life insurance premiums had been reduced.

"That's because medicine can now cure so many diseases," he said.

"Name one disease medicine can cure," I said.

"There's lots of them."

I replied, "Tell me one disease that medicine can cure. We have more diabetes than ever before, more cancers, more strokes and medicine has become the fourth leading cause of death in this country."

Contrary to popular belief, people are not living that much longer today than they were one hundred years ago. According to *Sugar Busters*, a book written by three specialists in internal medicine and a Fortune 500 executive, a fifty-year-old person in the year 2000 would only live eighteen months longer than a fifty-year-old person in the year 1900. The big difference in longevity is predicated on the fact that infant mortality has been reduced by hygienic conditions and better birthing procedures, the pasteurization of milk, sanitary sewers, safe water supplies, modern housing, smaller families, the refrigeration of foods, the elimination of rats, mice, and insects, and the modern processing of foods.

If you doubt the above statement may I suggest you visit a local cemetery and read the tombstones of all the people who died in their eighties, nineties, and hundreds. In the year of 1900 if a child died in infancy and their grandfather died at 100, the life expectancy of those two people was fifty years. Yet, neither of them died at age fifty.

Medicines are designed to stimulate or inhibit the functions of the human body. They are not designed to cure. Is high blood pressure curable? No, you have to take medicine the rest of your days. There's still no cure for the common cold or the flu. Yet millions of people are given worthless antibiotics when the doctor knows perfectly well that antibiotics do not cure viral diseases.

Fifty million people in America now fall in the category of being hypertensive. When I went to school in the 1950s normal systolic blood pressure was established as 110 plus half your age for a male and 100 plus half your age for a female.

Every few years pressure is brought to bear on health organizations to lower the levels for normal blood pressure with millions of people now needing drugs to control their pressure. Millions of those same people could lower their blood pressure by exercising, losing weight, taking hot baths, using biofeedback, taking potassium and magnesium supplements and reducing salt intake.

The University of Arizona School of Pharmacy reported in 2001 that Americans spend seventy-five billion dollars on drugs each year and seventy-six billion dollars to treat the side effects of those drugs.

Dr. Charles Mayo, one of the famous Mayo brothers of medicine stated, "Nine tenths of the surgery in the United States is unnecessary and the other one-tenth should be performed by someone who was merely qualified to do surgery."

American surgeons do five times as many hysterectomies, back surgeries, and mastectomies as European doctors do.

In the early seventies *U.S. News and World Report* had an excellent article about life expectancy in the United States. They reported that people who lived in South Dakota had the greatest life expectancy of those in any state in the United States. They also pointed out that South Dakota had the fewest number of doctors in proportion to the population of that state. Since that time the state has had a marked increase in physician population and now has fallen far out of first place for longevity. It certainly wasn't the climate that caused them to live longer back in the seventies.

Antidepressants and suicide

My suspicions when I first read and heard about the Red Lake, Minnesota School shooting was, "I'll bet drugs were involved." According to news articles about the massacre of innocent students, Jeff Weise, was taking sixty milligrams per day of Prozac.

Students high on prescription drugs were also responsible for the Columbine, Colorado and Kip Kinkel's Oregon's murderous killings and wounding of scores of innocent victims.

Over the last several years a total of eight of the school shootings were performed by students on antidepressant drugs (Prozac, Paxil, and Luvox).

The side effects of those drugs include an increased tendency to commit suicide, serious allergic reactions, and conversion to mania in bipolar disorders. Five additional shootings have taken place since 1998 but those records are sealed. Why?

The shootings have resulted in nearly one hundred dead or wounded students. Every parent's nightmare today. Could it happen at your school? If my memory serves me correctly one of the shooters murdered his parents, slept in the same room with their corpses and then shot up his fellow students the following day.

These drugs now are carrying a warning label that they increase the risk of suicide.

Ritalin's effect on our children

The drug Ritalin is frequently used to help relieve the hyperactivity of children with attention-deficit disorder. In the spring of 2005 news sources reported that researchers had discovered a link between the use of Ritalin and cancer.

The children did not actually have cancer, but after three months, every child receiving Ritalin treatment had a three-fold increase in chromosomal abnormalities associated with cancer.

The study was conducted by the University of Texas and the MD Anderson Cancer Center in Houston.

Other studies show that a side effect of Ritalin is failure by children to grow to normal stature. Six to ten million Americans use Ritalin. As expected, the manufacturer defends the use of the drug.

Aspirin isn't harmless

Acetylsalicylic acid (ASA): Americans spend billions on it and gobble it up in tablet form. Commonly known as aspirin, it is America's most widely used drug, both singularly and in combination with many prescription and patent medicines.

Unfortunately, most people think that aspirin is a harmless drug, though it is not. It may injure the stomach (sometimes severely), interfere with the absorption of several vitamins (especially C, K, and folic acid), and pose a special risk for pregnant women and patients with bleeding disorders such as ulcers.

Aspirin leads all over-the-counter drugs in causing adverse reactions requiring hospitalization. It is the major cause of childhood poisonings, as indicated by a recent National Safety Council report claiming that 400 children died in one year from ASA ingestion, many from just one or two tablets.

In 1981 I authored an article warning that children suffering from influenza or chickenpox, if given aspirin, could develop Reye's syndrome (RS). This hazard was described in a publication released by the FDA as far back as 1978, and between that year and 1985, over 1,500 children died from RS. I personally believe that the aspirin manufacturers deliberately suppressed this vital information.

Aspirin given to pregnant women may interfere with the absorption and metabolism of folic acid in the fetus and result in such deformities as cleft palate or spina bifida in their offspring.

ASA has no effect on viruses or bacteria. It won't help a cold or the flu, nor will it shorten the duration of either. In fact, according to recent scientific evidence, it may prolong recovery. Aspirin used in combination with alcohol is even more damaging to stomach membranes. Not only can it cause heartburn, dyspepsia of the stomach, discomfort, nausea and vomiting, it is also responsible for ulcers with perforation and bleeding of the stomach mucosa and membranes, and gastrointestinal hemorrhage. Considering the fact that ulcers may lead to cancer of the stomach, this is certainly an ominous reaction.

Dr. Robert Schuller, pastor of California's Crystal Cathedral landmark church, reported on his Sunday morning broadcast that he had struck his head on a car door during a visit to Holland years ago. He took four aspirin for the resulting headache from the injury; this thinned his blood and caused a stroke, requiring two brain surgeries to correct a hemorrhage in his brain. Those four aspirin nearly cost him his life!

> Dr. Robert Schuller of the Crystal Cathedral took four aspirin after an injury. Those four aspirin nearly cost him his life!

Although commonly prescribed for heart attack prevention in the United States, a *British Medical Journal* report claimed that ASA was taken daily by 22,000 MDs, with no reduction in cardiac arrest, but with an increase in strokes. Patients with high blood pressure should not take aspirin because of the propensity of this latter occurrence.

It has been estimated that one aspirin causes a loss of one teaspoon of blood from the stomach membranes. Continued and prolonged use may elicit enough blood loss to cause iron deficiency anemia. Taken in combination with other drugs such as anticoagulants, ASA may cause severe liver damage and possibly death. It may also depress kidney function in certain patients.

Aspirin blocks the enzyme cyclooxygenase, used in forming prostaglandins, which are "hormone-like" substances crucial in the alteration of blood vessel diameter. They also elevate body temperature when infection is present, play an important role in the clotting of blood, and protect the stomach membranes from excess acid formation. Interfering with prostaglandin production may alter our body's natural response to inflammation and delay the healing process.

ASA may cause or aggravate asthma. An allergic reaction to aspirin can also lead to other breathing problems. Large doses of the medication are also correlated with deafness and tinnitus (ringing in the ears).

One question is puzzling this author: Why are aspirin and other over-the-counter (OTC) drugs called anti-inflammatory drugs, when their most serious and common side effect is inflammation of the stomach? If these drugs are not safe to take when a woman is pregnant, why are they safe to ingest when she is not pregnant?

A number of OTC drugs interfere with the absorption and metabolism of Vitamin C, which is necessary for the manufacture of collagen, present in cartilaginous material and necessary for joint repair. Therefore, when one takes OTC drugs for inflamed joints, they're actually causing damage to the tissues they're trying to repair.

Another result of aspirin ingestion may be hives. This is not limited to ASA, however; people who are allergic to aspirin can also be allergic to ibuprofen, ketoprofen, and naproxen.

ASA shares a common ingredient with corn salve, which burns the flesh off your feet. The only time aspirin should be taken is when one has a "corn" between the ears!

The future of drug misuse

According to an Associated Press article, the U.S. Government will target the use and abuse of pain medicines, sedatives, and stimulants. Well, it's about time. The excessive consumption of these dangerous substances has exploded during the last ten years.

Doctor shopping and acquiring large supplies of prescription drugs has come to the forefront lately. Prescription drugs rank second only to marijuana as being the most misused by both adults and teens.

Internet availability of Oxycontin and Vicodin will come under surveillance of federal authorities.

FDA commissioner Mark B. McClellan is quoted as saying, "No medicine is completely safe."

A Michigan study of high school seniors found they used twice as much Vicodin as cocaine, ecstasy and meth.

Critics of the government's actions claim they will result in causing doctors to undertreat pain.

Do you really believe that your headaches or back problems are caused by a deficiency of Aspirin, Tylenol, or Motrin in your body? If you believe that, I'd like to sell you some seashore property in Montana.

Chiropractors maintain that pain is the body's warning sign. It implies that a vertebra or other joint might be out of place, pinching nerves and interfering with normal function.

When the oil warning light on your car goes on, do you put an aspirin in your crankcase?

The drugs I've mentioned do not correct the cause of your problem. They merely cover up the symptoms, exactly like the ostrich putting his head in the sand so he doesn't see the lion that is attacking him.

It wouldn't be so bad if those over-the-counter drugs did no harm. Instead, they are loaded with serious side effects. *The Los Angeles Times* printed a report a few years ago that twenty percent of all dialysis patients got on dialysis from taking ibuprofen products such as Motrin, Advil, Nuprin, and Aleve. There has been a three hundred percent increase in kidney failure cases since 1989, when ibuprofen products were introduced.

At the Hagen Clinic we frequently find that patients taking ibuprofen products have blood and albumin in their urine, indicating kidney damage.

During September 1998 I attended a chiropractic meeting in Minneapolis at the Hotel Sofitel. Next door to our meeting, the Mayo Clinic was conducting a meeting on liver transplantation. One of their sessions was on liver transplantation made necessary because of Tylenol ingestion. I asked if I could attend that session and received permission to do so. I probably took more notes than the other two hundred medical doctors combined.

I learned that 70,000 liver failures occur each year and that 35,000 result from the ingestion of Tylenol and other over-the-counter drugs. You may be especially susceptible if you use alcoholic beverages with Tylenol or are on anti-convulsive medication. Don't they sell Tylenol in most bars?

A pharmacist friend of mine told me that we had a college student in our area who had died two years previously. The student had a bad cold and was taking a cough medicine with Tylenol in it. He was also taking an antihistamine with Tylenol, plus Tylenol for his aches and pains. The combination of those three medicines cost him his life.

You can avoid most medications by correcting the cause of your problem instead of treating your symptoms. Every function in your body is controlled either directly or indirectly by your nervous system.

Your nerves lead from the brain down your spine and thirty-one pairs of spinal nerves exit from the spine and lead to all your cells, tissues, and systems. Chiropractic care is predicated on restoring the spine to proper alignment, normalizing your nervous system and restoring function naturally.

Doesn't that make sense to you? If you want to stop living on pills that may make you worse, call an alternative practitioner.

Remember, when your spine's in line, you'll feel fine!

Some pills give you more than you ask for

Medicines often bring on unintended consequences. You hear the possibility of some of the negative results of taking a pill when you watch or listen to an advertisement for a specific drug. Nausea, vomiting, thirst, weight gain or loss, weakness, headache, and dizziness are just a few of the most common "side effects," as these unintended consequences are called. More serious ones include an increased risk of stroke, heart disease, liver failure, and even death.

For example, let's look at the arthritis drug Remicade. Researchers have found that people taking this drug have three times the risk of lymphoma as those who do not take the drug. Patients being treated with Remicade are also more likely to be susceptible to tuberculosis, and blood tests have shown a lower white blood count and fewer platelets in the blood.

Try not to get shots

Children are forced to submit to 22 immunizations before they enter school even though, according to statistics, 95 percent of those diseases had disappeared by 1970, long before childhood immunizations were mandated.

The vaccines contain mercury, aluminum, formaldehyde, and many other poisonous substances. As a result, there has been a 300 percent increase in autism and asthma.

America is the only nation I know of that requires males to be immunized for rubella, a relatively mild form of measles.

Almost every case of polio reported since 1978 was caused by the polio vaccine. Salk said the Sabin vaccine was no good, and Sabin said the Salk vaccine was no good. I think they were both right.

Children dying from measles

The Associated Press reported in March of 2005 that hundreds of children in Nigeria died from measles after a series of measles vaccination campaigns.

You've probably heard about Vioxx. Users who took this drug were promised relief from arthritis. However, the drug came with side effects that no one wanted: heart attacks, heart failure, chest pains, blood clots, serious bleeding, and death. The FDA has recalled the drug. My question is, "Why was it ever approved?"

We're always hearing that there's going to be a flu epidemic. Then we hear there's going to be a shortage of the vaccine. Finally the flu strain is announced, usually named after some Pacific Ocean country.

Let me ask you a question: "If the flu is a new strain, how can the antigens of that particular strain be in the vaccine? The answer is easy. Flu immunization is a multibillion-dollar business.

Unfortunately, after frightening the entire population with a campaign of fear about influenza, people marketing the most recent vaccine stand back and watch folks become sick with the flu anyway. Many will die from the vaccine.

My neighbor and his wife recently got the vaccine, and then they both got the flu.

This happens thousands of times every flu season.

A newspaper headline on November 18, 2004, announced that the FDA had failed to heed repeated warnings about the contamination of the flu vaccine manufactured by the Chiron flu vaccine plant.

According to the article British health authorities found widespread contamination of the vaccine with dangerous bacteria over the past five years.

FDA commissioner Lester Crawford denied making a mistake in allowing Chiron to continue manufacturing the contaminated vaccine.

Twenty problems were found during the 2003 inspection of the Liverpool plant. Similar problems were also found going all the way back to 1999.

Flu vaccine recipients are frequently told it's impossible to get sick from the vaccine because it's made with a killed virus. Contamination explains why people have sometimes violent reactions including death, paralysis, and hospitalization from the vaccine.

Mercury in childhood vaccinations

In 2001 a law firm in Dallas, Texas, filed the first known civil case against a major drug manufacturer for mercury poisoning in children receiving one or more of thirty childhood vaccinations containing the substance.

Mercury is the only metal that is liquid at room temperature. It is also the most toxic element on earth after plutonium. You can swallow elemental liquid mercury without suffering ill effects because it does not pass through the cells lining the stomach or intestines. However, when exposed to room temperature, some of the mercury vaporizes. If you breathe the vapor, the mercury moves directly to your bloodstream and brain. Depending on the dose and other factors, you may soon feel the ill effects of the vapor, and it may lead to a life-long disorder or a fatal illness.

I am concerned about mercury in the vaccines we continue to give our children. It comes to them in a chemical compound called thimerosal that contains 49.6 percent mercury by weight. It has been used since the 1930s to keep vaccines from spoiling while in transit and in storage. If you've ever watched the nurse fill a needle with vaccine, you probably saw the needle penetrating the rubber stopper on the vial with the vaccine inside. Even though the needles themselves are sterilized and free from germs, bacteria forming on the rubber stopper can contaminate the needle. Thimerosal prevents this from happening. Unfortunately, the mercury in thimerosal is sufficient to cause serious developmental and nervous system problems, especially in the unborn children of pregnant women being vaccinated and babies and young children receiving routine vaccinations.

Research points to high levels of mercury from thimerosal as a cause of the increase in autism in children. Thimerosal is also linked to other central nervous diseases including learning disabilities, Alzheimer's, multiple sclerosis, fibromyalgia, lupus, chronic fatigue syndrome, arthritis, depression, and bipolar disorder.

While most childhood vaccines made today are free from thimerosal, the federal agencies responsible for our health and safety, including the CDC and the FDA, took nearly two decades to recognize the risk shown in numerous scientific studies and take steps to prevent it from worsening.

Does immunization prevent disease?

Everyone recognizes the fact that you can create immune bodies in a patient by injecting either active or passive vaccines into their systems. However, because of a toxic reaction to the vaccines, many times we are killing more people by immunization than we are saving.

The polio epidemic in the early 1950s was a terrible medical catastrophe for American citizens and for people around the world. In 1952, 52,000 cases of polio were reported in the United States, and no vaccine was present. In the following year, 1953, 32,000 reported cases occurred; still no vaccine was available. Then in 1954 there were 20,000 reported cases of polio and there was still no vaccine.

In 1955 the polio vaccine was invented. Eleven million out of 55 million susceptible people were immunized. The number of cases of polio in 1955 was 18,000.

Scientists found that the polio vaccine was ineffective in many cases, so people that had the polio vaccine continued to acquire poliomyelitis. At first they said that you needed one immunization and then two and then three and then four and then an annual booster. Polio continued to decline. Was this the nature of the disease or was this due to the polio vaccination?

Since 1978, almost all polio in the United States was caused by the vaccination, with either a sibling or a parent of the vaccinated patient acquiring the disease. One wonders if polio might have been like scarlet fever for which no vaccine was ever made and the bubonic plague and other diseases for which no vaccines were ever developed. In my opinion there has never been a time when half of the susceptible people in the

United States of America have been properly immunized against poliomyelitis. I have never had a polio vaccine nor have any my children or grandchildren.

> During the fifties more people died of tetanus shots than died from tetanus.

During the fifties more people died of tetanus shots than died from tetanus. In fact it was mandatory that the person administrating the shot had to have a shot of epinephrine on the table in case the patient went into anaphylactic shock.

Dr. Mercola at Mercola.com reports in an article about vaccination that according to the morbidity and mortality reports of The Metropolitan Life Insurance Company that 95 percent of the contagious childhood illnesses had disappeared before 1970 before mandatory vaccination was legislated.

The reason for the disappearance of those diseases did not occur because of antibiotics or vaccination. Almost all of those diseases were caused by viruses and antibiotics don't work against viruses. Remember, there were no vaccines for scarlet fever, mumps or chicken pox (until recently), or tuberculosis. Those diseases disappeared because of hygienic and sanitary improvements in our refrigeration of foods, pasteurization of milk, furnaces, garbage disposal, elimination of rodents, and sewer systems.

Although we supposedly lost half our flu vaccine supply in 2004, we had one of the lowest incidences of flu that year. Every year the vaccine companies and government agencies scare us with the prognostications of a severe flu epidemic and they usually name it after an Asian country. Many of my patients who submitted to the vaccine have had severe reactions and have been hospitalized for many days. We lost one of our medical doctors in Sioux Falls, South Dakota, last year immediately after receiving a flu vaccine.

I've been collecting data on vaccinations for fifty years. If you would read all of the data, you would avoid immunizations.

The mortality and severe reaction to immunizations are grossly under reported. Estimates in health care publications have stated that only two percent of the vaccine reactions are reported. MDs are unlikely to accept responsibility for vaccine reactions.

The only immunization my children ever received was after my youngest child had a third of his mouth bitten off by a German Shepherd when he was five years old.

The tetanus bacillus is found in sheep and horse manure. It is an anaerobic bacterium. It lives in the absence of air. Because of the fact that he was bitten by a dog on a farm that had several horses I did not object to the doctor administering a Tetanus shot. Unfortunately he went into anaphylactic shock and they had to use a defibrillator to revive him.

Many of the catastrophic diseases of mankind have been solved by hygiene and sanitation. Consider the fact that barely 75 years ago we did not have sanitary sewers and water systems. Many farms had their septic tank above their well. There was no pasteurization of milk, a process that destroys bacteria. There was no eradication program for mosquitoes, rodents, insects, and disease bearing animals.

I give full credit to the eradication of many diseases to vacuum cleaners, refrigeration of foods, restaurant inspections, food inspections, and higher nutritional standards.

By the time a senior student graduates from high school he has received twenty-seven recommended immunizations. With the injection of all of these foreign substances into our blood stream is it any wonder that we have a 300 percent increase in cancer, asthma, autism, and other auto-immune diseases?

I remember a statement from a prominent physician fifty years ago that stated that he had never seen a case of cancer in an unvaccinated person.

The last case of smallpox in this country occurred in 1947. Due to the persistence of health officials mandating and requiring vaccination of our youth we had four hundred deaths from vaccines for the smallpox, before it was finally eliminated from childhood vaccine requirements. One person who contributed greatly to the cessation of mandatory smallpox vaccination was Dr. C. Henry Kempe, who noticed that many children were dying from the vaccine reaction, but no one had the disease. It took him ten years to stop this insane practice.

> It took ten years and 400 deaths from smallpox vaccine before Dr. Kempe and others were able to stop this insane practice.

There was a health report called the Philippine Report in the early part of the twentieth century that reported, after vaccinating every person from one to six times they had a very severe outbreak of smallpox in the Philippine Islands, and sixty percent of the people that had been vaccinated contracted the disease. It was also noted in that report that on Mindanao, where the Muslim religion prevented inoculations, there was only a ten percent incidence of the smallpox disease.

In fact, the last outbreak of smallpox among American people was in 1947 when one hundred forty-seven GIs stationed in Korea came down with smallpox. All of these GIs had been vaccinated one or two times prior to being sent to the Korean Peninsula.

Forty thousand first responders have been vaccinated for smallpox. Nine hundred vaccine adverse reactions have been reported with one death and seventy-five cases of heart inflammation. Congress has given power to public health officials to force vaccination whenever the government declares and "imminent" public health emergency. One wonders how many severe unreported reactions and deaths might have occurred from these 40,000 vaccinated guinea pigs. The majority of vaccine reactions go unreported.

I've had people cough on me almost every day of my practice. My patients that get adjusted regularly many times are the only ones in their family that do not get sick when the rest of the family does.

An experiment was conducted in one of our chiropractic colleges years ago showing a marked increase in the WBCs after adjustments were made. When you adjust the cervical spine of a person with a cold, sinus trouble, or allergies it always loosens up their nose immediately.

Dr. Robert Mendelson, a prominent pediatrician and columnist in over four hundred newspapers was criticized by his own profession for condemning the practice of immunization. He pointed out that we were killing a lot of people trying to save a few.

Many years ago the school nurse from the Iowa town where we were living called and informed me that my children had not been immunized against smallpox. I replied to her that "Nor will they be."

"Well, they will get smallpox and die."

I asked her if all of the other kids had been immunized.

"Yes, indeed," she assured me.

"Then how are my kids going to get smallpox if the vaccination program works?"

She didn't say anything. I continued. "Are you aware that hundreds of children have died from the smallpox vaccine and that no one has contracted the disease since 1947?"

"I am not aware of those circumstances," she replied.

"What age are you?"

She said, "I am fifty-three years of age." She told me she had an immunization against smallpox as a three-year-old.

"The smallpox vaccine supposedly lasts only three years, I said. "What protected you the other fifty years?"

Again, she had no answer.

William Boyd's *Textbook of Pathology* reported years ago that the whooping cough immunization was disappointing and that whooping cough resembled a viral type disease instead of a bacterial disease. The bacillus pertussis vaccine of the DPT shot is capable of causing deleterious effects.

For more information on the vagaries of immunization I would suggest that you order a copy of *A Shot in the Dark,* by Harris L. Coulter. The book is available on the Web as well as through some health food stores and major book distributors.

In his book, *How to Raise a Healthy Child in Spite of Your Doctor,* Robert Mendelson, M.D., included a chapter on problems with immunizations, beginning with the following statement: "The greatest threat of childhood diseases lies in the dangerous and ineffectual efforts made to prevent them through mass immunization."

> "The greatest threat of childhood diseases lies in the dangerous and ineffectual efforts made to prevent them through mass immunization."
> —Robert Mendelson, M.D.

He also said in this chapter that there are "significant risks associated with every vaccine and numerous contraindications that may make it dangerous for the shots to be given to your child."

Are these risks unknown—like the risk of being hit head-on by a delivery truck on your way home from work tonight? Not at all. Dr. Mendelson continues, "While the myriad short-term hazards of most immunizations are known (but rarely explained), no one knows the long-term consequences of inject-ing foreign proteins into the body of your child." Even more startling, he says, "there is a growing suspicion that immuniza-tion against relatively harmless childhood diseases may be responsible for the dramatic increase in autoimmune disease since mass inoculations were introduced. These diseases include cancer, leukemia, rheumatoid arthritis, multiple sclero-sis, Lou Gehrig's disease, lupus, and the Guillain-Barre syn-drome." Dr. Mendelson also suggests that vaccination may be a cause of Sudden Infant Death Syndrome (SIDS).

Speaking in 1988 at a health conference in Sioux Falls, South Dakota, Dr. Mendelson reported that the World Health Organization had blamed the AIDS epidemic on reactions to the smallpox vaccine.

He further stated that they expected an outbreak of smallpox in the African continent; therefore, health experts mandated a large vaccine program.

The vaccine for smallpox is performed by injecting a nee-dle saturated with puss from the infected belly of a cow into the shoulder of the recipient fifteen to twenty times. The practitio-ners of the vaccination program were supposed to sterilize the needles between each vaccination. Failing to do this, they spread AIDS from person to person until now twenty million people have died from this disease. Many more will die of it over the next half century.

The National Vaccine Information Center (NVIC) strongly criticized the May 18, 2004 report on autism and vaccines issued by the Immunization Safety Review Committee of the Institute of Medicine (IOM). A national press release from the center claimed that the report seriously jeopardized IOM's credibility to conduct independent, unbiased analyses of vaccine risk.

NVIC also released a letter written by NVIC President, Bar-bara Loe Fisher, to the National Academy of Sciences on Decem-ber 18, 2000 expressing concern about the ideological and professional conflicts of interest of members of the Committee.

The IOM report rejected emerging clinical and biological mechanism evidence, including experimental studies in ani-mals, demonstrating a causal relationship between neuroim-mune dysfunction and vaccination. But it was statements issued by the IOM Immunization Safety Review Committee calling for an end to research into vaccine-associated autism and suggesting that the cost of caring for autistic children should be eliminated from future cost-benefit analyses of thimerosal (mercury) risks, that prompted NVIC to brand the report a case of "political immunology."

The NVIC is made up of many parents of vaccine-injured children. The Institute of Medicine receives funding from the pharmaceutical industry, government agencies and private foundations to provide "independent" analyses of scientific and public health policy issues.

The medical profession has mandated a mandatory vaccination for children. If they required adults to be immunized for all of these various diseases you would have an outpouring of resistance from the adult population. Because children are not vocal enough to stop the madness, this practice will continue under the pretext of helping to prevent disease in children.

Reporting on the vaccination system

Mandatory reports of adverse events from routine vaccinations are supposed to be reported to the VAERS which stands for Vaccine Adverse Events Reporting System. Some interesting information was found in the Centers for Disease Control's *Morbidity and Mortality Weekly Report* dated January 24, 2003. A total of 128,717 adverse events were reported between 1991-2001. Fourteen percent of all reports described serious adverse events including death, life-threatening illness, hospitalization, prolonged hospitalization, or permanent disability.

This is a voluntary or passive reporting system reported by care givers, patients or others. This method of collecting information leads to under reporting, according to the article. Only one percent of adverse events are reported by patients or their parents. Doctors fail to report or minimize the reactions because of the fear of litigation.

Although many patients tell me about their children's severe reactions and hospitalization they are unaware of the doctor reporting the episode.

The influenza vaccine is known to increase the risk of Guillain-Barre Syndrome.

From September 1, 1998 through December, 1999, 121 reports of intussusception occurred in infants that received the Rotavirus vaccine (RRV-TV). Manufacturers subsequently ceased manufacturing the vaccine.

The reporting system received 1,580 reports of adverse events between March 1, 1995 to December, 2001.

An article appeared in Dr. Ted Koren's newsletter February 8, 2006, reporting on studies of flu vaccine recipients between 1970 and 1980 by Hugh Fudenberg, M.D. a world-renown immune specialist. The research showed a tenfold increase in Alzheimer's disease among persons receiving a flu shot for five years in a row after age 55. The cause of the increased risk is evidently due to mercury, aluminum, and formaldehyde present in the vaccine. Dr. Fudenberg spoke at the International Vaccine Conference in 1997 and has published 850 peer review articles. He is the thirteenth most quoted immunogeneticist in our time.

Flu shots can cause the flu

In a speech in 1988, Dr. Mendelson described attending a wedding. When he asked where the four grandparents of the bride and groom were, he was told that they were all ill, suffering from after-effects of a flu vaccine.

It has been my experience that many of my patients who have had a flu shot got the flu, and a number of people have been hospitalized as a result.

Many years ago I received a shipment of a thousand vials of flu vaccine sent to my office by mistake. It was supposed to go to the medical clinic across the street from my office. Upon opening the package I discovered a brochure describing the side effects of the vaccine. The list included meningitis, encephalitis, arthritis, anaphylactic shock (which is fatal fifty percent of the time), high fever, joint pain, and many other side effects.

The only flu immunization I have ever taken was when I was in the service and I almost died after receiving that vaccine. I told that story in the first chapter of this book.

Several years ago Harry Smith interviewed Dr. Bob Arnot, CBS medical director, on national television. Dr. Arnot advised everybody to get a flu shot as soon as possible. When Harry

Smith asked him if he had had a flu shot he replied that he had not. That ought to tell us something about the flu vaccine.

One wonders when we have a new flu each year, how the vaccine would be able to protect Americans from that particular viral species. We are great for naming influenza for Asians. We have the Asian flu, swine flu, the Chinese flu, the Japanese flu, the Hong Kong flu, and more.

Swine flu all over again

There is a striking similarity between the recent Avian Flu scare and the Swine Flu fiasco that happened thirty years ago. Swine Flu was a disease that never happened for which a vaccine was manufactured with side effects that no one wanted. Many people died from the results of that vaccine program and thousands of people were afflicted with Guillain-Barre's Syndrome (paralysis).

Billions of dollars in damages were paid out to the thousands of patients who suffered disabling and fatal side effects from the vaccine that vaccine manufacturers cleverly foisted upon our government by asking the government to assume responsibility and liability for the unpredictable side effects of that vaccine.

Dr. J. Anthony Morris was fired from his governmental virology job for saying that the Swine Flu posed no danger to the public.

I knew that Swine Flu was a farce when news media claimed this was the same flu that killed millions of people, including my uncle, in 1918. The only way you can observe a virus is with an electron microscope. According to my encyclopedia the electron microscope was not invented until 1937, so apparently no one saw that 1918 virus.

Fifty-five million Americans were gullible enough to stand in line waiting for this vaccine which was manufactured with toxic substances such as mercury, formaldehyde, and aluminum present in the vaccine. Three people in Omaha, Nebraska, were vaccinated, walked a few feet and died. The health experts called this a coincidence. Have you ever seen three people die suddenly at a football or basketball game?

Every summer health experts predict that we are just around the corner from an upcoming pandemic (worldwide) flu outbreak. They delight in naming these suspected epidemics after Asian cities or countries such as the Hong Kong or Singapore Flu. Everyone is encouraged to run to the doctor as soon as possible to receive the latest vaccine. No one explains to the public how this new virus has been captured and is readily available in the current vaccine.

My cousin's wife is still in a wheel chair since receiving a flu shot almost forty years ago. My only flu shot was given to me courtesy of the USAF on Guam. The next day they carried me to the dispensary. The diagnosis was influenza and I was advised that I needed a flu shot.

Dr. J. Anthony Morris was sent by our government to the Carolina Islands in the South Pacific to learn why the natives escaped the flu epidemic that occurred in 1918. While there our government initiated a flu vaccine program. Guess what?

Following the vaccine program they had a influenza epidemic on the Carolina Islands. When he got back to the States and reported what happened he was ordered to destroy his records. Look up Dr. J. Anthony Morris on Google. You'll find some very interesting information about vaccines.

I also suggest that you look up an e-mail dptshot@sbcglobal.net for information about a book by Marge Grant entitled, *A Stolen Life*. In a conversation I had with Mrs. Grant she told me she fears that with all the attention focused on the Avian Flu that congress will grant permanent immunity to doctors and drug companies for any and all injuries caused by vaccines. Senator Bill Frist who received over $800,000 in campaign contributions from drug companies for his last election has tried several times to introduce and pass this type of legislation.

An article finally appeared in the national news in 2005 stating that after thirty years of subjecting our senior citizens to yearly vaccines very little benefit occurred.

Although doctors are supposed to report adverse effects of vaccinations in both adults and children they seldom comply even though our government has a Mandatory Vaccine Reaction Reporting System. Experts estimate that only about two percent of the reactions or deaths are reported. Every year dozens of my patients tell me how sick they were and several were hospitalized following their immunization. A doctor in Sioux Falls, South Dakota, died following a flu shot last year. His lips swelled up and burst. A tracheotomy was performed but it was too late to save him.

The author on vaccine related injuries has suggested that perhaps the marked increase in Alzheimer's Disease is caused by the mercury and other toxins in all of the vaccines the elderly are taking.

Doctors, hospitals and pharmaceutical companies make a fortune off of all the visits and reactions related to the annual flu scare They won't make a dime off of me. If you're ill you're liable to have a severe reaction from the vaccine. If you're healthy you don't need one.

The supposed swine flu epidemic occurred years ago. The federal government provided liability for this vaccine program because the drug companies refused to accept responsibility for adverse reaction in patients. Thus far the government has spent close to $30 billion on injury cases. There are only three documented cases of the disease that was the target of the shot.

You may have heard the swine flu vaccination described as a program invented for a disease that nobody had with a vaccine with side effects that nobody wanted.

Because of the swine flu fiasco, Dr. J. Anthony Morris, formerly with the U.S. Food and Drug Administration and the National Institutes of Health, became a severe critic of vaccines. He stated that the swine flu vaccine was unsafe, that no one had the disease, and that we should not proceed to immunize the fifty-five million people who subsequently were immunized. For his candor he was fired from his job and defamed in the national press.

It was my pleasure to appear at the Iowa state capitol objecting to the mandatory implementation of vaccine programs for school children. Dr. Morris succinctly voiced his objection to mandatory immunization at that hearing, but to no avail.

Listen to Marge Grant

Marge Grant is the author of *A Stolen Life* and the mother of Scott Grant, who suffered severe irreversible brain damage as an infant in 1961 from childhood vaccines. The profound vaccine injury rendered Scott a lifelong non-ambulatory, spastic quadriplegic that created indescribable challenges for him and his entire family. It literally gave rise to Marge becoming a vaccine heretic and pioneering a nation-wide vaccine safety movement.

Marge is co-founder of Wisconsin Citizens For Free Choice In Immunization, an organization of committed parents who successfully petitioned their state legislators in 1979 and 1980 to change the law to allow parents the "freedom to choose" whether or not to have their children vaccinated before entering school.

She and her husband Jim founded the Wisconsin parent organization, DPT-SHOT, the acronym for "Determined Parents To Stop Hurting Our Tots."

Because of her son's profound vaccine injury and her intense endeavors to keep informed of crucial vaccine issues, Marge made forty trips to Washington, D.C. to repeatedly testify before the United States Congress. She served on the Advisory Commission on Childhood Vaccines (ACCV), to represent children who have suffered vaccine-related injury or death. She also served on the National Academy of Science, Institute of Medicine's Vaccine Safety Forum, for several years.

You can learn more about Marge Grant's struggle with the politics of vaccinations at her website, www.dptshot.com.

Some notes about vaccination

Here are some quotes and facts I've picked up about the dangers of mass vaccinations in our society.

- W. B. Clark, M.D. observes. "There was never a time when over ten percent of the world's population was ever vaccinated for smallpox."

- A quote from George Bernard Shaw: "More people die from vaccinations than the disease they were designed to prevent."

- Every single vaccine can cause encephalitis or meningitis.

- One percent of vaccinated kids wind up with autism.

- Vaccines contain aluminum, mercury, and formaldehyde.

- Your body is a whole lot smarter than your doctor.

- The U.S. is the most vaccinated country in the world, but we are one of the sickest nations.

- Only one in fifty vaccine-damaged children is reported.

- Crib deaths were unheard of before vaccination became mandated.

- Bubonic plague, typhoid fever, and tuberculosis, and scarlet fever disappeared without vaccines.

- Vaccines are not studied in combinations.

- A five-pound infant and a sixty-pound child may receive the same dosage.

- Interference and damage to the nervous system from a vaccination may seriously damage the immune system.

- You were born to be healthy.

- Forty-five vaccines by age six, seventy-four before graduating from high school.

Watch what you eat

You're an unusual person if you haven't been barraged with diet after diet to help you lose weight or obtain an ideal nutritional balance.

The Atkins low-carb diet plan seems to be regaining popularity although some people are not able to tolerate the high concentration of protein in the diet. One study by the North American Association for the Study of Obesity found that a low-fat diet is more successful than a low-carb diet.

The idea behind the Atkins plan is to induce a condition called ketosis. If the body doesn't have enough carbohydrates in the system, the body burns other substances for energy, including the ketones in stored fat and protein. Weight loss results. Many experts believe it was the fact that dieters on the Atkins plan cut their consumption by 1,000 calories a day and not the abundance of protein or the lack of carbohydrates that is responsible for phenomenal weight loss by some participants.

It is much better to follow a balanced eating plan with no sugar or white flour and an abundance of vegetables. One study found that men consuming twenty-eight servings of vegetables per week had a 35 percent lower risk of prostate cancer than those who ate fourteen or fewer servings per week. The results were even better (a 41 percent lower risk) for men who ate three or more servings of cruciferous vegetables—cabbage, cauliflower, broccoli, Brussels sprouts—a week. Doctors now know that the male prostate gland contains high levels of zinc. Patients dignosed with prostate gland disease are usually found with lowe levels of zinc. For many women with female disorders, copper levels are abnormal.

It is also safer to lose only one or two pounds a week. Pounds lost rapidly almost always come back, and serious illness can result from poor nutrition.

The book, *Sugar Busters,* advises readers to avoid red and white potatoes, white rice, corn, popcorn, cornmeal, corn bread, carrots, beets, white bread, sugar, products containing refined sugar, cookies and cakes made with sugar, and refined white flour. The authors do not recommend specific foods or describe how to combine them to keep your blood sugar at moderate to low levels.

Weigh right and feel good

Two-thirds of our adult population is obese. One-third of our children are obese. I cannot think of one advantage of obesity. I can think of dozens of liabilities.

We could cut our health care costs by at least fifty percent in this country if every one was at his or her ideal weight. Obesity is the leading causative factor in heart attacks, strokes, diabetes, arthritis, and kidney disorders.

We should begin losing excess weight by removing fast food and pop machines from our schools and serving nutritious foods. Skim milk instead of chocolate, chicken instead of burgers, salads and vegetables and a piece of fresh fruit for dessert should be the rule. Drinking water instead of soda would reduce appetites and cut way down on their caloric intake. A can of soda may contain ten to fifteen teaspoons of sugar. Children today are drinking more soda than water.

Potato chips, by the way, are not considered a vegetable.

Eat better, live better

Want to live longer and decrease your risk of heart trouble? Jean Carper told readers of *USA Weekend* in February, 2005, to consume nearly a pound of fruits and vegetables, two and a half ounces of almonds, five ounces of wine, one clove of garlic, three and a half ounces of dark chocolate, and four ounces of fish— daily!

Almost nothing you do has as much of an impact on your long life as your diet. Most people dig their own grave with their teeth. Two-thirds of our adult population in the United States is obese. That statistic alone signals a tragic consequence in life expectancy tables during the next generation. Death from heart disease, cancer, and diabetes are expected to skyrocket in the future. After years of anticholesterol drug therapy heart disease continues to be the major killer of mankind.

One third of our school children are obese. I went to a beach in Wisconsin this summer and was astounded at the large number of corpulent high school children swimming there. When I graduated from high school fifty-eight years ago we had one football player that weighed over two hundred pounds. Today the linemen weigh closer to three hundred pounds.

Almost all American adults are deficient in several nutrients. If you use alcohol, antacids, aspirin, birth control pills, caffeine, diuretics, laxatives, steroids, estrogen, or sweat a lot, chances are you're deficient in several nutrients.

One reason for widespread nutritional deficiencies is that most doctors are poorly trained in nutrition and so lack the ability to identify and treat nutritional disorders. Dr. Emanuel Cheraskin, author of many published articles on nutrition, says the average doctor knows only a little more about nutrition than his secretary—unless his secretary has a weight problem, and then the secretary knows more than the doctor does.

A nutritional balance is extremely important during pregnancy. Pregnant women endanger their fetus by using alcohol, antacids, aspirin, coffee, colas, or tobacco because all of these substances rob the body of folic acid. Deficiency of folic acid heightens the risk of a baby born with cleft palate and spina bifida.

We weigh too much

Obesity is now a $100 billion problem when we consider the amount of money spent on diets, exercise equipment, loss of time on the job, and the treatment of disease related to obesity.

We are a nation of unsurpassed wealth, a high standard of living, a plentiful food supply—and a paucity of proper information about what constitutes a healthy diet. Instead of considering the facts, we give in to the bombardment of television ads extolling the virtues of processed, radiated, and demineralized foods as well as foods laced with fat and sugar.

Beer isn't food and causes harm to the body and brain, but is a leading promoter of most athletic events.

I have helped many of my patients lose weight with proper diet and exercise. I also recommend the following:

- Stay away from fat people. They don't want you to succeed in maintaining a healthy weight. Alcoholics who want to give up drinking won't get encouragement from other alcoholics. Cigarette smokers who want to quit should hang out with non-smokers or they'll never stop smoking.

- Remember: You can't eat what you don't have in the house. Throw out or give away high-fat, high-sugar, low-fiber foods you might be tempted to eat. Stay out of restaurants noted for their high-fat specialties. Look for restaurants with heart-healthy menu items.

- Chew your food thoroughly. Aunt Martha was right when she told you to chew each bite twenty-two times. Digestion begins in the mouth. Your teeth are designed to cut, tear, and grind your food into smaller particles and then mix those particles with the digestive juices secreted by your salivary glands.

- Enjoy your meals. Dining should be a long-lasting, pleasant, socializing experience. The French, Italians, and Spaniards live longer than we do and have fewer obesity problem. It's not unusual for these people to spend three hours in the evening dining in a relaxed social setting. Most of us Americans spend only a few minutes eating all three of our standard meals.

- Take smaller bites. It's a fact that obese people tend to take large bites and swallow their food without proper mastication. Cut your bites down to one-third the size you're used to. Lay your silverware down on the table between bites. Don't chew with your mouth open; besides being ill mannered, it will mix your food with air and give you gas.

- Drink more water. You should drink eight to ten glasses of water every day—more if you are doing a lot of physical activity, and the temperature is high. Don't drink water during your meals or you will dilute your digestive juices. Water balances your body chemistry and helps to satiate your appetite. Don't count coffee and cola drinks as part of your normal water intake.

- Prefer fresh before frozen and frozen before canned in selection of fruits and vegetables. Only a few foods such as the carrot and the tomato are enhanced nutritionally by cooking. For most vegetables, heat destroys many vitamins and some minerals.

- Cook meat to kill organisms that could infect your body. Cooking will usually prevent infection and maintain most nutrients.

- Broil, boil, and bake rather than subject your body to high-fat deep-fried foods.

- Avoid eating before retiring at night. Most cholesterol is manufactured by your body at night.

- Avoid all-you-can eat buffets and remember that meat portions should be the size of the palm of your hand and the thickness of a slice of bread.

- Take a good vitamin and mineral supplement. I suggest buying these at a health food store where you can usually get good information about what is best for you.

- Avoid carbonated beverages. Carbon dioxide is a waste product eliminated by our lungs. Does it make sense to drink a waste product?

- Avoid artificial sweeteners. More research is needed on the toxic effects of these chemical compounds, although it has been reported that excessive consumption of diet drinks has apparently caused some pilots to have convulsions.

- If it tastes good—don't eat it. It's probably bad for you!

Hypoglycemia

Hypoglycemia is defined as an abnormally low blood sugar level and is a very common condition. For persons with diabetes, low blood sugar occurs as a result of too much insulin injected. That is why diabetics usually carry an orange or a sugar lump with them to counteract the effects of hypoglycemia. It is also found frequently in the general population.

Reactive hypoglycemia following a meal is the most common type. It usually occurs two to four hours after eating. The symptoms include headaches, light headedness, fainting, weakness, trembling, rapid beating heart, excessive hunger, excessive sweating, confusion and visual disturbances. Difficulty in standing and walking may also occur. One unusual diagnostic sign is lack of hair on the outside of the calves of the legs.

The secret of avoiding hypoglycemia is to eat several small meals two to three hours apart, which incidentally is a good idea for anyone wanting to lose weight. If you suffer from hypoglycemia chances are you will be overweight. Those patients that have the mentioned symptoms should carry fruit to work with them and eat a piece of fruit mid morning and mid afternoon. Soups are also good if available for lunch. By all means avoid white sugar and white flour.

Remember the French paradox

We just don't get it. The French are known for their rich diets. They love croissants, brie, and pastry. At every meal it seems they revel in fatty foods such as butter, cream, foie gras, pastry, and cheese. And yet only seven percent of the French adult population is obese. They eat three times as much saturated fat as Americans do, but are only one-third as likely to die of a heart attack.

What is going on?

Through the years many explanations have been offered to explain the "French paradox." The only one that makes sense in explaining their trim weight is that the French consume fewer calories than we do, but what about heart disease? How can they eat so much saturated fat and still have a low rate of heart disease?

We now know that the answer is probably related to portion size as a major cause of total calories consumed. Research shows that the average serving size in an American restaurant is twenty-five percent larger than in comparable eating places in France.

Some medical writers believe that the French advantage won't last much longer. Today they are eating more and more hamburgers and french fries—they call it the "McDonaldization" of the French diet. It's just a matter of time until they catch up with us and begin suffering the same high rates of heart disease.

Food labels can't always be trusted

When you consider buying a packaged food product at the grocery store, you may glance at the food labels to see how many calories are involved and other nutritional numbers that are important to you. An interesting study by the FDA found that one out of ten nutritional labels had at least one inaccuracy and that this was an excellent record.

The law concerning food labels is not violated unless an item is more than twenty percent off. The government also allows a ten percent margin of error for its laboratory tests to determine label accuracy.

Add to this the fact that what is printed on the label doesn't necessarily indicate what is in the product in the package. For example, the label by one doughnut vendor, according to an ABC News report in May of 2004, said its carob-coated doughnut had just three grams of fat and 135 calories. It actually was a chocolate doughnut with 18 grams of fat and 530 calories. Another label on a bag of chocolate chips claimed there were no carbs in the product; actually it had 14.2 grams. Blueberry muffins probably contain artificial blueberry-flavored bits, and no blueberries at all. Many products listing milk, fruits, or vegetables as ingredients do not contain them.

The best way to combat inaccurate labels on processed foods is not to buy them. You can make your own food at home much more healthfully—and at less cost—than by buying packages of highly processed, nutrition-deprived, calorie-rich foods.

The Hagen Color Diet

My program for weight control is entitled "The Hagen Color Diet."

The basics of this program identify the foods that are bad for you by color. To follow this program you will avoid the "six whites," the "six browns," and the "six yellows." Here they are:

The six whites

1. White sugar
2. White flour
3. Salt
4. Milk (except skim)
5. White rice
6. Cigarettes

The six browns

1. Cola drinks
2. Coffee
3. Chocolate
4. Gravy
5. Meat
6. Tea (except herbal teas)

The six yellows

1. Lard
2. Egg yolks
3. Butter
4. Oleomargarine
5. Cheese (except "hoop" or Farmer's cheese)
6. Oils and fats

If you change your diet and eliminate all of these foods, you'll also eliminate most of the high-calorie fat that can compromise your weight problem. Add a walking program of two to three miles daily, and you should be able to develop a healthy body and extend your life expectancy.

Why the 'Six Whites' are bad

The "six whites" are cigarettes, sugar, salt, white flower, white rice, and milk (except for skimmed milk).

Avoid them.

The average American consumes more than 150 pounds of sugar each year. I consume very little, so someone must be eating my share. A ten-ounce can of soda may contain ten teaspoons of sugar. Would you let your children put ten teaspoons of sugar on their breakfast food? Dr. Mercola at www.Mercola.com has a list of more than 100 reasons why you should avoid sugar.

What about salt? In the process of manufacturing, salt is heated and chemicals are added to keep it from caking. Sea salt is all right to eat in moderation. I have not had a salt shaker on my table for twenty-five years, and my blood tests show high levels of sodium.

White rice and white flour are made from grains that have had as many as 26 nutrients removed. The manufacturers add six of the cheapest nutrients back into the product and have the audacity to call it "Enriched." It should be labeled "Devitalized." Animals are fed the fiber from the grains, and I've never seen a constipated cow. About eighty percent of the adult population has occasional problems with constipation. No wonder. When you mix white flour with water, what do you get? Paste.

The reason I advocate skim milk instead of whole milk is because of the fat content and high cholesterol levels in whole milk.

'The whiter the bread, the quicker you're dead'

The above slogan appeared on the sides of bakery trucks in Milwaukee, Wisconsin. White bread lacks nutrients removed during the milling of the flour. Much of the fiber and as many as 26 nutrients have been removed. A half dozen are added back into the white flour. Remember that white flour and water makes paste. No wonder so many people are constipated.

Did you ever see a constipated cow? I grew up in Wisconsin and worked my way through school on dairy farms. It's a good idea not to stand directly behind a cow, especially if they've just been turned out on green grass. A diet without white flour obviously keeps cows from being constipated.

Throw away your salt shaker

Nearly thirty years ago I threw away the salt shaker. Every year I have a blood test and a hair analysis. My tests are always high in sodium and chloride.

Salt is ubiquitous. It's in most of our foods. In more than fifty years of practice I've only come across two patients who were deficient in salt. Both of them were taking medicines that washed the salt out of their bodies.

Salt is a combination of sodium and chloride. The government's Recommended Daily Allowance (RDA) for sodium in adults is 500 milligrams. The average American consumes about 3,500 milligrams of sodium every day.

Adults also require 750 milligrams of chloride, which is part of stomach acid, or HCL. It helps regulate the osmotic pressure of the cells of the body. Sodium along with potassium is involved with muscle contraction and expansion as well as nerve stimulation, making minerals more soluble and absorbable. Chloride also aids in body reflexes, improves blood and lymph and is involved in the excretion by the body of carbon dioxide.

Scientists estimate that excessive consumption of salt causes 150,000 premature deaths each year. The Center for Science in the Public Interest has sued the FDA trying to force them to restrict salt consumption to one teaspoon (2300 milligrams) per day and

> Excessive use of salt causes an estimated 150,000 premature deaths per year.

even less (1500 milligrams) per day for African Americans. Most Americans consume two to five times that amount.

I went to our pantry while writing this article and looked at several items. For Bush Best Baked Beans, I found that half a cup contains 680 milligrams of sodium. Seven Tostitos 100 percent white corn chips contained 120 milligrams (but who stops at seven?). Two tablespoons of unpopped popcorn contains 460 milligrams of sodium, raisin bran cereal, three-quarter cup, 250 milligrams, and a half cup of canned kidney beans, 400 milligrams.

Always read the labels for sodium content. Buy products with no salt added to the original food. Rinse canned foods such as beans, tuna, and chicken. Don't consume salted nuts, bacon, ham, salted fish, sharp-flavored cheese, pickles, cold cuts, high salt breads, and fast foods. Certain milk products also contain high levels of salt.

The Pritikin Longevity Center recommends avoiding foods with more milligrams of sodium in a serving than calories. An excellent video on labeling can be ordered from www.Pritikin.com entitled, "Health Food v. Healthy Food" and "Going Nuts? The Facts on Fats!" Jeff Novick, MS, RD, LD/N, is the author and narrator.

I recommend sea salt because it is richer in natural elements. The salt in your salt shaker contains sodium, chloride and residual amounts of other chemicals. Sea salt has 84 natural elements that we need to be healthy.

The 'Sugar Busters'

Three medical specialists and the CEO of a Fortune 500 company in New Orleans have joined forces to author a book with the title, *Sugar Busters*.

The book places the blame for America's problem of obesity on the excessive consumption of sugar. Americans consume more than 150 pounds of sugar per person every year. The authors aren't concerned about calories. They recognize that especially refined sugar causes a marked elevation of a person's production of glucose. More glucose in the system causes the pancreas to produce more insulin in order to metabolize the glucose. This signals the body to store fat.

The authors of *Sugar Busters* state that not using sugar will lower cholesterol levels, help achieve ideal weight, give more energy, and prevent many chronic diseases. The "sugar busters" program aims to eliminate or reduce the intake of sugar while balancing nutritional needs in a positive manner. More than 200,000 attest to the principles in this book, which includes a 14-day menu program and recipes.

Lower your cholesterol levels

Cholesterol is not a fat and is not related to saturated fats. It is a sterol found in every living cell in the body and helps hold cell membranes together. It is a part of steroids, hormones, bile acids, and sex hormones. Most of our cholesterol is produced in the liver, with only about twenty percent coming from the food we eat.

In my opinion the drug companies that sell anti-cholesterol drugs have conspired to constantly lower the normal level in order to sell more drugs. Today the public is advised to maintain a total cholesterol level of 200 or less. Every time the normal levels are reduced, millions of potential users are created.

The best way to lower your cholesterol level is by a proper diet. Eliminate the saturated fats from your diet. Avoid coconut and palm oils and margarine. Increase your exercise level and a number of nutrients are helpful in lowering cholesterol. The Pritikin Diet has been very successful at lowering cholesterol in program participants. Look up www.Pritikin.com.

The Multiple Risk Factor Intervention Trial (MRFIT) found that men with a cholesterol level of 240 or more were 2.2 to 3.6 times more likely to die from heart disease than those with levels under 200.

What is the cost per month? How about the side effects? Rhabdomyolysis, a wasting away of muscle is a severe, sometimes irreversible side effect of statin drugs. Crestor now requires a label concerning muscle wasting. Baycol has been withdrawn because of side effects, including deaths. Other potential side effects include liver damage, increase in breast cancer, severe constipation, flatulence, hemorrhoids, dyspepsia, and abdominal pain.

Cholesterol drugs also lower your CoQ10 level, a coenzyme that increases your energy levels and does prevent heart attacks. Cholesterol drugs also rob your body of all of the fat soluble vitamins (ADEK), folic acid and niacin.

I have read numerous articles stating that between fifty and sixty percent of all heart attack victims have normal cholesterol levels.

Trans-fatty acids

Trans-fatty acids are the bad fats. They gum up your arteries and veins. They raise your LDLs, the bad cholesterol, and lower your HDLs, your good cholesterol.

They occur as a result of hardening of polyunsaturated oils that are hydrogenated to transfer liquid fats into solid foods. Margarines are good examples. Avoid eating any food that is hydrogenated or contains animal fat. The lower the fat content of your diet, except for small amounts of essential fatty acids, the healthier your diet.

On the August 19, 2005 *Today Show,* Dr. Karen Mechels of the Harvard School of Medicine reported that eating one serving per week of French fries increased the risk of breast cancers in females by 27 percent. The increase is apparently due to the ingestion of saturated fats and trans-fatty acids.

Is alcohol bad for you?

The authors of *Sugar Busters* point out that a glass of wine has fewer calories than a piece of white bread. Medical journals have reported that a glass or two of red wine every day is good for your health. The wine should not be taken on an empty stomach but preferably after you have eaten food with fat or protein in it. Residents of France, Italy, and Spain consume large quantities of wine with their evening meals yet have lower levels of alcoholism and heart disease than Americans do.

Beer, on the other hand, has a high content of maltose, which is fattening. It should be avoided as should any substance ending in "ose" because they are a form of sugar. Lactose, fructose, sucrose, and maltose are examples.

If you choose to drink alcoholic beverages, be careful. Excessive alcohol consumption has dire consequences, and many people seem to be "programmed" by the way the circuitry of their brain is wired to become addicted to alcohol.

Fast foods

The majority of foods at fast food restaurants are loaded with too much, fat, salt, sugar, protein, and calories. Another problem with fast food is we eat the food too fast. Because we don't take time to chew it, the food enters our alimentary tract without adequate chewing. Eating it too fast, drinking too much soda with it and combining the wrong types of foods for proper digestion ends up causing stomach problems.

No wonder we have acid stomachs, and eighty percent of the adult population has elimination problems.

If it's advertised on TV, it may not be good for you

I've noticed that most of the foods that are advertised on TV are not nutritious. Most cereals are loaded with sugars. Saturated fat products are heavily advertised on TV. Sodas that contain ten to fourteen teaspoons of sugar per serving have been responsible for children drinking more sodas than water each day. Carbonated sweetened beverages increase damage to dental enamel eleven-fold.

Orange juice contains 180 calories per glass. It's better to eat one orange that has only sixty calories but is more filling. Skim milk should be preferred over whole milk even though it is not often advertised as being better for you. Meat should be eaten sparingly with the fat trimmed off. Sugar products should be restricted but instead are highly touted by the sugar industry.

Sprayed food can be toxic

I remember reading in a farm magazine about apples that were sprayed over thirty times before they were harvested for human consumption.

Years ago chickens and cattle were injected with stilbestrol. Then it was discovered that there was an increased cancer risk for people that ate the Stilbestrol-treated chickens. Now chickens cannot be treated with this dangerous product.

People were worried that it was still being injected in cattle, but Dr. Wise Burroughs of the State University of Iowa assured the news media that it was safe for treating cattle. Two weeks later the *Iowa Des Moines Register* reported that Dr. Burroughs was the developer of stilbestrol and that he and Iowa State University had received more than a million dollars in royalties.

This is another good example of what happens when the fox is hired to guard the hen house.

Dead doctors don't lie

Joel Wallach DVM, ND, has become a mighty advocate of simple health practices. Forty-five million tapes of his talk, "Dead Doctors Don't Lie," have been sold worldwide. He discovered that most human and animal diseases are caused by nutritional deficiencies and developed numerous vitamin and mineral preparations made with organic or plant-based sources. Dr. Wallach endorses chiropractic and other natural healing methods.

Dr. Wallach was nominated for the 1991 Nobel Peace Prize for his discovery that cystic fibrosis was associated with a selenium deficiency in animals. He did not receive the award because members of the prize committee did not accept his findings. Today his ideas remain highly controversial.

We know that iron-rich minerals are absorbable in small percentages. Ferrous sulfate, for example, can be absorbed at a one percent rate, ferrous fumarate at seventeen percent, and the iron in black strap molasses at a much higher percentage.

- Ninety-nine percent of people in America are deficient in minerals.

- Copper deficiency causes gray hair and aneurisms.

- Selenium deficiency leads to age spots.

- A chromium deficiency is associated with diabetes.

- A shortage of calcium can cause arthritis, spurs, fractures, insomnia, muscle cramps, twitching, and PMS.

- Most people require mineral supplements in addition to the food they eat because farmers only add N_2 (nitrogen), phosphorus, and potash to the soils.

Happy families

A family, whether it's a couple in their 90s or a bustling family with half a dozen youngsters scrambling through the house, should be a haven of peace for its members.

The most urgent need of a newborn infant is bonding, the development of an intense attachment between the baby and the baby's parents. Without bonding, the child may not fully develop self-esteem and social skills. Studies of orphaned children show that babies who were well-fed and clothed but never held, rocked, or touched in a loving way failed to develop normally. If severely deprived of human touch, brain damage and even death will result.

We don't lose our need for touching and social contact with other human beings when we leave childhood behind. Adolescents deeply involved in asserting their independence appreciate a hug or a pat on the back from a parent. Marriages grow in satisfaction through the years in proportion to the happiness a husband and wife experience in each other's company. And in old age, being around friendly people and participating in life in a meaningful way are highly effective ways to postpone, alleviate or prevent many forms of senility and debilitating illness.

Happy marriage

We have half as many divorces in our society every year as we do marriages. Half of our marriages today end in divorce. There is good news for those that remain happily married. They will live an average of seven years longer than unmarried persons.

Most marriages wind up in divorce when husbands and wives lose the romance in their marriages. Remember, God didn't put romance in marriages, He put romance in people. It's up to you to keep the romance alive. A marriage in Kansas City ended years ago when the wife filed for divorce because her husband squeezed the toothpaste tube from the top instead of from the bottom.

A doctor stated several years ago that he advised young women getting married that they should keep the husband's tummy full and his prostate empty. A good sex life assures fidelity. A survey recently showed that couples that averaged sex twice weekly greatly enhanced their longevity. Maybe you should make a copy of this page and paste it on the bathroom mirror.

A few ideas to assure a happy married life:

1. Be hearty in your approbation and lavish in your praise.

2. Never put each other down.

3. Have a weekly date.

4. Remember important dates.

5. Hug a lot. It's healthy.

6. Don't criticize, condemn or complain.

7. Share hobbies together.

8. Read good books on marriage that aren't written by old maids or bachelors.

9. Take yearly vacations together.

10. Hang out with happily married people.

11. Worship together.

12. Support each other when times are tough.

Keep the romance in your marriage

God doesn't put romance in marriages; he puts romance in people.

Whether you're the husband or the wife, take your spouse out on a date regardless of how many years you've been married. My dentist used to double date with his father who was in his 90s. They all had a great time going out for dinner and seeing good plays, movies and concerts.

Wives love flowers. Bring them to her spontaneously. You don't have to be in the doghouse to have an excuse to surprise her with flowers. Husbands love tools and gadgets. Make a note the next time he mumbles about a tool he needs and buy it—or give him a gift certificate to his favorite hardware or computer store.

While we were raising our family of six robust children, my wife and I would often get a baby-sitter for the week end and go to a large city where we would play tennis, eat in nice restaurants, stay in a good hotel, and take in a movie.

Have a good sex life

Science assures us that sex is good for us. Studies show that people with a good sex life have better health and live longer. I refer without exception to a monogamous sex life: one man, one woman. The sex life of a homosexual or a prostitute does not lead to longevity.

We winter in California, and I am always shocked at obituaries in the newspaper of people in their 30s, 40s, and 50s dying of AIDS. Last year I saw a report that Palm Springs, California, has the highest incidence of venereal disease in the country, especially of syphilis. What a tragedy. Syphilis cannot be cured. If given antibiotics, the person with syphilis may suffer brain damage because the antibiotics can drive spirochetes out of the blood stream into the nervous system and brain. A significant number of incurable mentally ill persons are there because of complications of syphilis.

Pregnancy is not a disease

Too many doctors treat pregnant women as if they are suffering from a life-threatening disease instead of going through a natural biological process.

The bad advice begins when women are advised to watch their weight rather than being told what to eat. The mother-to-be should be advised to get the vitamins and minerals she needs from food rather than from a prenatal bottle of pills. Liver, for example, is a better source of iron than is ferrous sulfate, which is absorbed at the miserly rate of one percent and usually causes constipation. Another good source of natural iron is black strap molasses.

> One out of three pregnant women suffer from malnutrition, and babies born to malnourished women may have serious health problems.

A federal survey a few years ago showed that one out of three pregnant women suffered from malnutrition, and this was attributed to advice from their doctors to try to keep from gaining more than ten pounds. Most doctors have little knowledge of nutrition, but the reality is that malnourished women have problems such as prolonged labor. Babies born to these women may have serious health problems.

Pregnant women should not smoke, or drink alcoholic or carbonated beverages. The excess phosphorous in sodas and other carbonated beverages depletes calcium from your bones, which are already stressed. They should also avoid smoking, alcohol, sodas (they rob the body of calcium), coffee, antacids, laxatives, sugar, and physical activity that causes excessive perspiration.

We advise our pregnant patients to stay reasonably active by walking, swimming, and performing yoga, but we do not recommend jogging or running. Sitting for long period of time should be avoided, and a visit to a gentle chiropractor should be scheduled if backaches result.

My daughter called me from London complaining that she was going to be delivered by a midwife or else it would cost her $10,000 for a medical doctor to deliver her child. I assured her that properly trained midwives have a better safety record than medical doctors because they will take time to comfort the expectant mother without inducing labor or performing a C-section. She was thrilled with her experience and delivered a ten-pound baby boy.

A few years later her doctor induced labor, and she was in labor for fifty hours. They very much advocate natural labor in England, but after that long in labor, I encouraged her to have a C-section. The baby boy weighed eleven pounds, three ounces.

Doctors in America rely too much on delivery tools and procedures such as forceps, episiotomies, ultrasounds, amniocentesis, induction of labor, anesthesia, drugs that prolong labor, fetal monitoring, and pain-killing injections that stop or prolong labor.

In spite of the new technical equipment and instruments used to deliver babies today, infant mortality and birth defects are increasing.

A University of Wisconsin doctor analyzed 2,000 births, nearly half of them at home, and found that home deliveries were far safer than hospital deliveries. Nevertheless, a midwife in my home state of South Dakota was arrested and fined for her work delivering babies at home.

My five siblings and myself were all born at home. My mother never had an episiotomy and was back on her feet within a day or two after delivery. We had no indoor plumbing, electricity, telephone, or furnace. The cost to my father for each delivery was $10 to $25.

Chiropractic during pregnancy

The pregnant woman has special health care needs that carry through to the delivery of a healthy baby. Chiropractic care has been a blessing for many women during their nine months of physiological stress.

My son Mark and I have treated approximately 350 pregnant mothers at our chiropractic clinic. We advise our patients to take vitamins months before conceiving and to avoid all medications while they are pregnant.

Chiropractic care is great for relieving morning sickness, backaches, headaches, constipation, sciatica, leg cramps, and even the "blues." The biggest benefit of all, though, seems to be a dramatic shortening of the delivery time. We seldom have a pregnant woman spend more than three hours in delivery.

You don't have to take medicines in order for chiropractic care to work. Even an aspirin can rob your body of folic acid, and a deficiency of this nutrient can cause birth defects such as cleft palate and spina bifida. Ibuprofin products cause kidney damage, and Tylenol may damage the liver.

The protrusion of the abdomen in the later stages of pregnancy causes an extra strain on the vertebrae of the lower back. If subluxated (misaligned) vertebrae were present before conception, back ache and leg problems usually develop as the unborn baby grows. Neck problems and headaches are common.

We have found that our expectant moms benefit tremendously from massage therapy. We have four massage therapists on our staff.

When chiropractic adjustments are needed on a pregnant woman, we use very gentle adjusting techniques. I cannot recall any patients whose symptoms worsened by their care at our clinic.

We recommend that all of our pregnant patients receive one adjustment a week during the final month of pregnancy.

During my wife's third delivery the doctor examined her and told her it would be at least eight hours before she would deliver. He told her he would go upstairs and sleep until the nurses woke him up for the actual delivery. As soon as the doctor left the room I adjusted her, and twenty minutes later our daughter Lisa was born. I can still remember the bewildered look on the doctor's face when he was called back for the delivery.

If you're wondering how in the world chiropractic can shorten delivery time, consider the fact that all muscles involved in the delivery process are controlled by nerves that originate in the brain, come down the spinal cord, and out between the vertebrae of the lower back and pelvis. Good spinal alignment, easy delivery. Misalignment, hard delivery. One of our patients delivered in thirteen minutes, and most deliver within three to four hours.

I read about a medical doctor in Chicago who testified in a chiropractor's antitrust suit against the American Medical Association that his pregnant patients who received chiropractic care before delivery gave birth in half the time of his other patients.

Suggestions for pregnant women

By taking the following precautions, women who are pregnant can avoid many of the problems women encounter during their pregnancy.

- Avoid all medicines during the pregnancy
- Avoid the smoking of cigarettes or the consumption of alcohol.
- Exercise daily with activities such as swimming, walking, and Yoga.
- Get plenty of sunshine but not a sunburn and no tanning treatments.

- Avoid all stress.

- Never sleep on your stomach. Sleep on your back or side. If you sleep on your side pull your knees up as far as comfortable and use two pillows. One under your head keeping your head straight with your spine and one between your legs to keep your pelvis lined up and to keep pressure off your bony knees.

- Take vitamins at least three to six months before becoming pregnant, and take a good calcium supplement (not Tums). The calcium product should also contain vitamin C, D, and K, magnesium, manganese, copper, and boron.

- Exercise daily with activities such as swimming, walking, and Yoga.

- Stop smoking. Smoking during pregnancy doubles the baby's risk of colic.

Breast feeding is the best

The best food for your newborn baby is milk from the breast of the mother. If you think about it, human milk is the best milk for human babies. There are about 4,000 different species of animals whose bodies provide milk for their young. The formula and chemical composition of milk for each type of animal is different. Cow's milk is formulated for baby cows. For your baby, human milk is the best. Choose breast feeding if you possibly can.

Of course if breast feeding is not feasible for you, cow's milk and other alternative milk products can be adapted, and your bottle-fed baby can grow up healthy.

Bottle-fed babies generally weigh more than breast-fed infants, but that isn't necessarily healthier. Actually, breast-fed babies take advantage of the antibodies in the mother's milk that help prevent disease. Some of the diseases that are prevented by breast milk include pneumonia, botulism, bronchitis, staphylococcal infections, influenza, ear infections, and German measles.

Scientists have also learned that mothers are able to produce antibodies in response to specific diseases in the environment. Mother's milk is custom designed for your baby.

Breast-fed babies have much better cholesterol profiles than enriched formula-fed babies do. This may statistically reduce their incidence of heart attacks and strokes later in their lives.

Reduce the risk of breast cancer

Cancer of the breast is now the second most common cancer found in females. Women past the age of forty account for 95 percent of breast cancer cases, according to 2003 cancer statistics, and affects five out of every 1,000 women in their late seventies. Deaths from breast cancer are exceeded only by deaths due to cancer of the lungs. One of every 100 breast cancers is found in males.

Billions of dollars are spent every year on examination and treatment of our female population to combat breast cancer. An untold cost is born by women who undergo the fear of confronting this disease even if they survive.

Twenty-five years ago Nathan Pritikin reported that breast cancer was rarely found in thirty-five Third World countries that were not consuming the high-fat diet we love so much in the U.S. As soon as the Western diet was introduced in these countries, the incidence of breast cancer increased.

The daily consumption of soy products such as tofu and tempe probably explains much of the lower incidence of breast cancer among Asian women. Many other risk-reducing foods can give women an edge in avoiding breast cancer, including the following:

- Cruciferous vegetables such as broccoli, cabbage, cauliflower, collard greens

- Foods containing folic acid, such as egg yolks, apricots, cantaloupe, avacados, beans, pears, cereals, oatmeal, artichokes, bananas, grapefruit, nuts, salmon, and chicken

- Vitamins A, C, E, and the minerals zinc and selenium have anti-oxidant benefits to prevent cancer

- Yellow and orange vegetables containing beta-carotene (Vitamin A)

- Lycopene in cooked tomatoes helps prevent prostate troubles in males and breast cancer in females.

- Dark green vegetables and all brightly colored fruits and vegetables are cancer-fighting foods

- Red wine and Concord grapes are rich in anti-oxidants

- Omega 3 oils found in cold water fish such as salmon, tuna, and sardines, as well as in walnuts and flaxseed oils may offer protection against breast cancers.

- Dark cherries are reported to have anti-tumor benefits in studies with lab rats

- Citrus fruits—whole fruit is better than juice from concentrate

- Dark green vegetables and all brightly colored fruits and vegetables

- Brown rice

- Double virgin oil in salads and in cooking

- Green tea has been reported to have anti-cancer benefits

- Spinach—a New York University study found that women who ate spinach twice weekly cut their risk of breast cancer by fifty percent.

- Taking vitamin supplements offers a low-cost means of reducing the incidence of many cancers that afflict humanity

High on the list of foods to avoid are those containing hydrogenated trans-fatty acids. This includes packaged cookies, french fries, and many commercially prepared snacks, often under the label "partially hydrogenated vegetable oils."

Nitrate-cured meats, alcohol, antacids, antibiotics, aspirin, birth control pills, cholesterol drugs, cola drinks, diuretics, estrogen, laxatives and sugar rob your body of excessive vitamins and minerals, setting you up to develop breast cancer and other diseases. Smoking, excessive sweating, and stress also make you more susceptible to breast cancer. Avoid pesticides and underarm deodorants containing aluminum. Red meat and dairy products contain a high percentage of fat as well as hormones fed to cattle to boost their growth.

Not surprisingly, obesity elevates the incidence of breast disease. Good old sunshine converts a chemical on your skin to Vitamin D, a vitamin you want to enlist on your side because it is anti-carcinogenic against both breast and colon cancer. We all need more sunshine—not sunburn, but healthy exposure to sunshine without jeopardizing our sensitive skin.

Breast feeding your child is beneficial not only to the child but to your mammary system as well. Daily exercise and a healthy weight as well as wearing breast-supporting garments that do not irritate tissue are all excellent practices for the woman who wants to be free from breast cancer.

Stay away from AIDS and HIV

The Centers for Disease Control estimates that 300,000 Americans are victims of AIDS or are HIV positive but do not know it. The good news today is that patients are living longer with AIDS than before. The bad news is that there are now more than a million persons with AIDS living in America. Almost half the victims are black. The incidence of sexually transmitted diseases, including AIDS, has increased by fifteen percent in women.

In 2004 AIDS was allocated far more money than sixteen other diseases that kill more people than AIDS. These include strokes, cardiovascular disease, cancer, diabetes, and Alzheimer's disease.

What disturbs many in the health care field is that most AIDS cases could be prevented by safe sex and the use of uncontaminated needless. Unfortunately, the general public winds up paying for the scourge of AIDS with tax dollars and higher premiums for health insurance.

Look for the good around you

A sage once said, "Your Attitude Determines Your Altitude." In more than fifty years of practice I've seen many people who suffered illness caused by their "Stinking Thinking." Your immune system and response to illness may be greatly affected by your attitude. My observation of people has supported this concept.

Look for the good in everybody and every circumstance. James 1, verse 2 in the New Testament says, "Count it all joy when you have trials and temptations." I cannot think of any trials in my life that did not produce something positive in the long run.

My good friend Charles "Tremendous" Jones, the author of *Life is Tremendous*, says every morning when he wakes up, "Lord, please give me some heart-rending problems to solve today." When he goes to bed at night he says, "Lord, you certainly answered that prayer in a hurry."

My mentor James W. Parker said, "What you see in the Universe sees you." Read *The Power of Positive Thinking* by Norman Vincent Peale, who lived up into his eighties; his wife is still active carrying on his work in her nineties. Make every circumstance in your life into a positive circumstance.

Terry Redlin, who has become one of the most famous artists in the world, lost a leg in a motorcycle accident in his late teens. Instead of moaning about his lot in his life he went to art school and became a great artist who has made millions off of his wonderful paintings.

All of the great people I've met and studied overcame adversity and did great things in their lives. You can, too.

Safe and healthy families

My youngest daughter swallowed some charcoal lighter fluid when she was three years old. We were lucky to save her life.

One of my colleagues finished some cabinets with a toxic sealer. The directions advised to be used only in a well ventilated room. It was thirty degrees below zero when he painted the cabinets, and he kept his windows closed. He became deathly ill shortly thereafter. He developed uncontrollable diabetes. The Mayo Clinic traced back his condition as having been caused by the sealer he had used.

We are surrounded by all kinds of unsafe chemicals that should not be inhaled or applied to our skin, dishes and utensils.

Be certain to read the labels on all the chemicals you have in your household or office. Place all poisons in locked storage cabinets or discard them properly. Throw away drugs and chemicals that have a stale date and dispose of them according to instructions.

Keep some charcoal tablets on your premises and any time someone swallows a poison get the charcoal in their stomachs as soon as is possible. If charcoal is not available, use milk. Don't induce vomiting when petroleum products are ingested. Call the Poison Control Center in your area.

Modern hazards

Just because it's been invented recently doesn't mean that a device is going to save lives—or even be safe to use. Every time a new medical tool or piece of equipment is announced, hopes soar that this will be the invention of the century. From babies born the size of an adult fist to workers burned beyond recognition in an industrial fire, the vision of no irreversible harm continues to play in our imaginations.

Common objects ranging from toss-out picnic plates to permanent structures such as the homes we live in and our places of business come packaged with surprising foibles and hazards. The astute reader will arm himself with information about dangers that lurk in everyday life and how to maximize protection against them.

Modern inventions

On June 17, 2005, the Guidant Corporation announced that it would be recalling nearly 50,000 defibrillators. Because of an "electrical flaw," almost 30,000 of them could develop short circuits and 21,000 might malfunction because of a computer error.

Two patients have died. Forty-five devices have failed. The defibrillator is about the size of a deck of cards and is implanted in the chest of the patients. Electrodes are attached to the heart and if the heartbeat is irregular it is supposed to shock the heart into action.

Vice President Cheney has one implanted in his chest, but his was manufactured by another company, so maybe he'll be lucky.

The FDA has advised patients that have received the faulty devices to consult with their physicians to see about replacing the devices.

Don't drive just any car

Automobile magazines publish a list every year of the safest cars to drive. Pay attention to that list. Drive a car that has roll-over protection and side as well as front air bags.

Once you've chosen a safe car, follow these suggestions for driving safely for years to come—

- Fasten your safety belt. It helps you sit up straighter and prevents you from being ejected from the car in case you have a roll-over accident.

- Place your headrest even with the top of your head to prevent whiplash injuries.

- Check your tires. Make certain they have sufficient tread and are rated for safety. Keep them properly inflated.

- Obey the speed limits and drive according to the road and weather conditions.

- Get out of your car at least once each hour. Walk around the car and get back in. It will save your back and may save your life by keeping you awake.

- Pull off and take a brief nap if you get sleepy.

- Don't drive for long periods of time without proper sleep.

- Don't drink when you drive.

- Don't smoke with the windows closed.

- Be courteous.

- When the weather turns bad, remember that you never really have to get there!

Avoid Teflon and artificial sweeteners

More and more articles are popping up on the Web con-demning the use of artificial sweeteners. Dr. Joseph Mercola, one of the most revered doctors in the field of alternative medicine, has lengthy articles concerning sweeteners such as Splenda, saccharine, and Aspartame (NutraSweet). Reports of pilots in the cockpits of airplanes suffering seizures from the diet drinks occurred several years ago. Splenda is actually made from sugar.

The sweeteners I recommend are honey, date sugar, Stevia, and maple syrup. Use them all sparingly because even these substances lower your white count. Avoid corn syrup as well, especially if you're squeamish about using genetically altered foods. Almost all corn syrup is made with genetically modified corn and processed with genetically modified enzymes.

You may have read in a health article that foods cooked, fried, or heated on Teflon surfaces may increase the risk of cancer. The culprit in Teflon appears to be the chemical, perfluorocotanoic acid, PFOA for short, a synthetic chemical used in the manufacture of advanced plastics including Teflon. A campaign has been launched to require the withdrawal of this chemical in manufacturing Teflon because of the alleged link to birth defects and other health problems.

New cars and new homes can be toxic

Many materials found in new cars and new homes may cause serious health problems for their proud new owners.

Volatile organic chemical compounds in plastics, vinyls, glues, paints, varnishes, wall coverings, carpeting material and sealers may cause headaches, dizziness, nausea, difficult breathing, or malaise, and some chemicals may be carcinogenic.

The "Sick Building Syndrome" has been known for years, but until recently specific health risks in new cars have not been identified. The Environmental Protection Agency issued a statement in 2000 that the air in new cars contains higher levels of vinyl chloride than does normal outdoor air because of vinyl chloride gas arising from new plastic parts and contributing to that "new car smell."

Formaldehyde is found in carpeting materials used in homes and cars and is regulated as a carcinogen by the Occupational Safety and Health Administration Agency.

What's the solution? Air out your new house or car before occupying it. Leave the windows open during good weather. Spend as little time as possible in either the house or car. You might also consider buying a used car or a house built more than six months ago.

Don't sit too long

Sitting is hard on the spine and the central nervous system, but lying down isn't the answer.

In one study, several Swedish medical students had needles connected to pressure gauges inserted into their intervertebral discs. Sitting resulted in a recording of 250 newtons of pressure whereas standing reduced the pressure to 150 newtons and lying down produced only fifty newtons of pressure.

Based on the research, doctors began putting bad back cases to bed for several weeks. A catastrophe resulted. Muscles withered, function was lost, and patients became discouraged.

What about electromagnetic fields?

You might be surprised to know that many electrical appliances you're using in your home give off electromagnetic frequencies or EMF.

The EMFs of certain electronic devices and overhead electric lines are thought to be deleterious to humans and animals when certain intensities are present. Many lawsuits have been filed against electrical companies for the death of livestock resulting from exposure to EMFs.

Almost everyone is aware of the fact that microwaves may cause problems with patients wearing pacemakers. I recently used a Gaussometer around several electrical devices in my new home. I found several high readings above the recommended tolerances of the manufacturer of the meters. The readings were pegged in front of the microwave even though it is a brand new make and model. The readings were also high in bedside alarm clocks and in front of TVs. It required ten or twelve feet distance from a TV before the readings were in the acceptable range.

My new Gateway computer showed a slight reading, which pleased me no end. I also perceived that I slept better when I removed the bedside alarm from the night stand next to my bed. If you use a microwave, immediately move far away after you start it. I would not recommend living near a power plant or under or near power lines. Fluorescent lights are not recommended by many health experts. We use full-spectrum lights in our clinics, and we designed the treatment rooms to be located on the south side of the clinic. This allows us natural sunlight to light and heat our rooms in the winter.

Don't use fluorescent lights

We use full-spectrum lights in our clinic. For information on the dangers of fluorescent lights, read Dr. John Ott's book entitled, *Health and Lights*. The use of fluorescent lights has been linked to attention deficit disorder (ADD) and leukemia.

Watch out for cell phones

No one appreciates the use of cell phones more than I. They've saved me many a trip. Almost everyone has one strapped to their belt.

The use of cell phones has been controversial ever since their invention. They have been accused of causing brain tumors, headaches, dizziness and other human aliments.

> **Worth a grin...**
>
> What is the difference between God and a medical doctor?
>
> God doesn't think he is a medical doctor.

I believe the earlier models poised a greater health risk than the most recent models. You'd probably be better off if you had a remote ear piece and microphone so that the device would not be next to your brain and ear. That would also certainly reduce your danger of death or injury from a car accident caused by distraction. My suggestion would be to use a regular phone whenever possible.

Stay back from your television screen

Your television screen gives off a tremendous amount of electromagnetic fields, and one hundred studies since 1990 blame EMFs for causing serious health problems. EMFs are now classified as a Class B carcinogen in the same category as DDT, dioxins and PCBs.

I recommend that you sit at least ten to twelve feet away from the tube. Children should not be seated directly in front of the set. You'll notice whenever you turn off your TV from the control on the set it creates a tremendous amount of static electricity on your hand and arm. Have a sleep control on your set so it turns off automatically if you fall asleep while watching it. Don't watch "spooky" TV programs" before retiring for the night.

You might want to invest in an inexpensive Gauss meter to measure EMFs in your home. Any reading above 0.5 mG is above "usual" levels, and the EPA has proposed a safety standard of 1.0 mG.

Natural cosmetics

There have been some alarming articles in national publications lately about dangerous chemicals used in the manufacture of cosmetics. I suggest to you if you are a woman, use discretion in the purchase of cosmetics. Several companies tout the natural ingredients of their products.

Wear clothing made from natural fibers

Fifty years ago while providing services in the Palmer College free clinics, we were required to wear a white nylon clinic jacket. Almost every day I left the clinic with a headache. I attributed the headache to the air conditioning in the clinic. Years later a well informed colleague told me it was most likely from wearing nylon. He advised me to wear clothing made from cotton, wool, silk, or leather. He even pointed out a passage in the Bible that said the same thing.

Take this test. Have someone hold their arm out parallel to the ground and then push down. Now put a piece of nylon over their body and the arm will go weak. I advise all professional athletes to wear cotton while participating in their sport. I also advise them not to wear metal around their necks. The same test will demonstrate that wearing metal will make the arm go weak. If anything weakens you it could affect your athletic performance.

Aluminum cans

Avoid eating and drinking foods or beverages from aluminum cans. I usually have a hair analysis each year. Whenever I drink sodas out of aluminum cans before taking the test, my hair samples show excess aluminum levels in my hair.

A University of Iowa School of Medicine study of patients who died from Alzheimer's disease showed that they had excessive levels of aluminum in their brains.

The British medical journal *Lancet* reported in 1989 that Alzheimer's disease was fifty percent greater in areas that had excessive aluminum levels in their drinking water. Post mortem or autopsy findings also found more aluminum in the brains of Alzheimer's patients.

Other aluminum products beside cans include deodorants, cookware made from aluminum, and food additives. Read the labels on all the foods you buy. Certain aspirin products and other pain medications, antacids, and shampoo products contain aluminum.

Live a long and satisfied life

Laughter and smiles

We are all aware that it takes far fewer muscles to smile than it does to frown. A smile makes you look younger and more pleasant. It enriches others without impoverishing you. At work, a smile goes a long way toward creating a pleasant environment. A pleasant expression increases your business and your rapport with all the people who surround you.

Norwegians are the second longest living population in the world. I believe it's because of their great sense of humor. Laughter does great things for your immune system. It raises the levels of your endorphins and enkephalins—hormones that strengthen your immune response.

Norman Cousins, the editor of the *Saturday Review,* wrote a wonderful book, *The Anatomy of an Illness*. Mr. Cousins was suffering from Ankylosing Spondylitis. This crippling disease literally welds your vertebrae together so that you lose your spinal mobility. Norman found that if he laughed a lot he felt much better, so he spliced old films of Abbot and Costello, The Three Stooges and other comedians together and watched them for hours. He also took huge dosages of vitamin C. He cured his disease by laughter. Yes, "Laughter is the Best Medicine."

A movie of his experiences was made starring Ed Asner as Norman Cousins. I remember a scene in the movie. A nurse came into his hospital room and asked for a urine specimen. Then she left the room. He noticed a pitcher of iced tea on the bedside table, so he filled the specimen cup with the iced tea. When she picked up the specimen cup she remarked how cloudy it was. Norman took the cup from her hand and said, "I'd better run it through again," and drank it down. The nurse fainted. Mr. Cousins went on to lecture at the ULCA School of Medicine until his death many years later.

Scientific papers have appeared lately extolling the healing qualities of laughter. One reported that laughter can dilate your blood vessels by twenty-two percent. Another stated that your blood pressure is

> Laughter dilates blood pressure and lowers blood pressure.

reduced by laughter. I noticed that my blood pressure fell by about twenty millimeters of mercury whenever I watched "Everybody Loves Raymond."

Hang around jolly, good natured people. Tell and listen to funny stories. Don't tell others your troubles, or who just died, or who's getting a divorce. Laugh at yourself and with others. I've noticed that the funniest comedians in television usually tell funny stories on themselves.

Dr. B. J. Palmer, the developer of chiropractic, gave millions of "Keep Smiling" cards away during his life time. Nothing disarms a stranger more than a genuine smile and a sparkle in your eye. A smile enriches others without impoverishing the giver. A smile tells others that you're healthy, happy, and well adjusted.

Never criticize, condemn, or complain

Three Cs you must remember and never do for the rest of your days: criticize, condemn, complain. On a positive thinking phonograph record Earl Nightingale produced years ago, he said, "You become what you think about." A good point, but not exactly true. If we became what we think about all day long, a lot of us guys would be women.

I had a patient years ago who couldn't wait to tell me who had just died, who was running around, who was getting a divorce, and who was having financial problems. I finally said, "Don't tell me the bad news. Tell me what is good that is happening in your neighborhood and to your relatives and friends."

Don't look for bad, sad, mad characteristics of different people you meet. Whatever you may feel inside, always speak kindly of your spouse, your children, and your relatives.

Socialize

It has long been known that bridge players are less likely to develop Alzheimer's than are people who do not play games or have interests that require exercising your mind. Worry warts or stressed-out individuals are 2.4 times more likely to develop Alzheimer's disease, which is a deterioration of the brain.

Your mind is like a muscle. It grows with exercise and degenerates with inactivity. The old adage, "Use it or lose it" applies perfectly to the human mind.

Worth a grin...
What accounts for the largest portion of health care costs?
Doctors trying to recoup their investment losses.

To make friends, be friendly. Some people who attend church look like they were baptized in lemon juice and took communion with vinegar. My friend James Parker said that some people are so cold that he couldn't warm up to them even if he was cremated with them. Another excellent way to socialize is to join the Lions, Rotary, Sertoma, or Kiwanis Club or similar organizations in your area. You'll have opportunity to contribute to your community and will be doing good for yourself at the same time.

Always be learning. I was the oldest in my graduating class when I received my second college degree at 51. I have taken courses in computers and have taken bridge lessons, tennis lessons, and golf lessons. I take fifty to one hundred hours of continuing education every year to keep me current in my profession.

The army has a great slogan, "Be the best that you can be." Ninety percent of us are not being the best that we can do.

Faith and expectations

Do you want to increase your life expectancy by seven years? Start going to church. People of faith live an average of seven years longer than unchurched people. Churched people are more likely to be satisfied with their lives, more likely to be sober, non-smoking, and less likely to be divorced. They are also less likely to commit suicide or murder, are involved in less crime, and are less likely to drive drunk. All of those are less likely to contribute to longevity.

Most people get what they expect out of life. If you expect to be successful, healthy, happy and well-adjusted you'll probably be successful, healthy, happy and well-adjusted. You get what you expect because you're already leaning in that direction. You need to have health goals just as you have personal goals for success.

I recently attended a seminar conducted by Mike Vance and Diane Deacon. They co-authored the book, *Think Out of the Box*. Vance reported that he had asked a Catholic nun who was in charge of 250 Catholic hospitals what her biggest problem was. She replied, "Pissing and Moaning." That's rather earthy language for a Sister, but it's a significant observation. Mike and Diane sell buttons with stamped out letters, "P&M." When your employees start P&M'ing, you hand them one of those buttons.

Wouldn't we all be a lot healthier if we quit P&M'ing?

Enjoy your work

If you want to live a long life, find an occupation or profession that you enjoy. My wife has never heard me say I've had a bad day at the office. If I told her I had a bad day she'd probably tell me what a lousy day she'd had and then we'd both be miserable.

My brother, Dr. David L. Hagen, has a sign in his office "Eight Hours of Fun." We're working, treating patients daily and still enjoying it, even though we're both up into our seventies.

Psychiatrists and psychologists have a very high suicide and divorce rate. While taking a behavioral studies course in college several years ago I asked the professor why people that study behavioral problems for seven to ten years should have trouble with their own life expectancy. He told me it was because they listened to patients describing terrible problems all day long. If they had sympathy and compassion for their patients they themselves became depressed. I then realized what a wonderful profession I had because I heard accolades all day: "I'm sleeping better." "I can play golf again." "I'm back to work."

Professional football players die at an average age of 52 because of all the violent collisions they have on the field. Football is hard on the spine, the brain, and the nervous system.

Worth a grin...

Bombeck's Rule of Medicine: Never go to a doctor whose office plants have died.

Workers who work in heavy industries are suffering from pollutants in their work environment. Coal miners have a lot of lung diseases. Asbestos workers have had a problem with asbestosis, especially if they smoked while spraying asbestos onto ships in an unventilated area. Heavy material handlers, truck drivers, and nurses have a lot of low back injuries.

Sedentary jobs are not necessarily good because sitting puts greater pressure on intervertebral discs than standing and moving does.

I've had the pleasure of studying ergonomics at the Harvard School of Public Health and am pleased to see their emphasis on the environment and health of the workers.

Be forever grateful

No matter how bad your lot in life may be, lots of people have it worse. I've been to Auschwitz and Birkenau, the infamous death camps in Poland. I have so much to be grateful for.

Thank God every day for another day of life. If you have a wonderful life, be grateful. If you have wonderful children, be grateful—and tell them you are. If you have a good job, be grateful. We live in a great country. Everybody in America should be grateful.

My mother died when I was five years old. I lived in seventeen homes and attended ten schools in the next eleven years. All I did was complain about my lot in life. then someone straightened me out at age twenty. I turned my life around and began concentrating on the positives instead of the negatives. Don't waste time on a pity party for yourself.

Compliment as many people as you can

Everybody remembers a compliment. Tell people something nice about themselves, and you will see them light up with the biggest smiles you have seen.

Read the book of Proverbs in the Bible for good advice on how to treat people. For example—

15:13 A glad heart makes a cheerful face; But an aching heart breaks the spirit.

15:18 A wrathful man stirs up contention, But one who is slow to anger appeases strife.

16:24 Pleasant words are a honeycomb, Sweet to the soul, and health to the bones.

18:24 A man of many companions may be ruined, But there is a friend who sticks closer than a brother.

20:7 A righteous man walks in integrity. Blessed are his children after him.

Hobbies

Everybody ought to have several hobbies. Bridge players have been reported to being less likely to have Alzheimer's or dementia. The same applies to people who do cross word puzzles. The more active an aged person the more likely he or she is to survive for a contented long life.

I've seen many people who quit working and without any hobbies survived only a short time. A good example is the occupation of farming. Farmers who move to town and don't have hobbies or keep on helping out on the farm don't last very long. Their wives survive much longer because they are still working.

I play tennis every day in the winter and golf several times each week in the summer. I try to play bridge frequently and use my computer daily. During the summer months I pick up cans along the road and still run my practice three days each week.

> **Worth a grin...**
>
> Doctor to patient: "Well, Mrs. Jones, I'm afraid you're not quite as sick as we'd hoped."

The Bible makes no provision for retirement. Several of my colleagues died the day they retired or shortly afterwards. For twelve years I traveled to foreign countries doing free clinics for the poor. We saw hundreds of patients each day. We worked far harder than we did at home, so when we got home we thought we were on vacation for the next fifty weeks. We also learned how lucky we were to live in America.

Two great books you must read

Two wonderful books that have been on the best sellers' list are *The Purpose Driven Life* by Pastor Rick Warren and *Your Best Life Now* by Pastor Joel Osteen. Buy those books, read them and then read them again.

Enthusiasm

Enthusiasm literally means to be with God. Dale Carnegie students are taught, "Act Enthusiastic and You'll be Enthusiastic." Any doctor will tell you that enthusiastic patients cooperate better and respond to care better than patients that act bad, sad, and mad.

Serving others

My personal observation is that people who spend a lifetime of serving others usually live long lives. This is true of missionaries who have gone abroad and lived amongst disease, pestilence, and abject poverty.

Helping others helps you. Be of service when you have no expectation of any personal benefit. Giving people a hand up is far better than giving them a handout. That's another way of saying that giving a person a fish will provide food for a day; teaching the person to fish can give them food for a lifetime.

Pets

Owning a pet keeps many senior citizens happy and healthy. They need to exercise their dogs and they benefit from going outdoors in the fresh air and from the long walks. Taking pets to nursing homes seems to perk up the senior citizens.

Love

Lather love lavishly. Love is its own reward. People in love have a spring in their step and a sparkle in their eye. Notice grandparents when they're around their grandchildren. They come alive.

Hugging therapy

Hug as many people as you can each day. My mother died when I was five. I can't remember being hugged after that for at least ten years. Now when I travel to foreign countries to do free clinics my only fee is a hug from my patients. I'm certain that some of those patients haven't been hugged in a long time. We both benefit from the hugs. It increases our endorphins. Studies have been done on the benefits of hug therapy.

I told a church group in Montego Bay in Jamaica that if they would start hugging others in church their membership would double. When I went back two years later they all greeted me as Dr. Hug, and their membership had doubled.

Do you know why they won't let people hug in some churches? It might lead to dancing. When a child is hurt and is crying, have you noticed that the moment you hug the child, he or she usually stops crying? If you want to keep your kids out of trouble, bring them up with hug therapy.

I teach hugging to doctors, wives, and receptionists. I tell them there are many kinds of hugs. For example, there is the "common hug" when billfolds kind of rub together. Then there is the "maternal hug" where the two huggers pat each other on the back like they are burping a child. Then there is the "Christian A-frame hug," where people stand as far as possible from each other while they are hugging.

A hug goes a long way when expressing bereavement and sympathy of all kinds. Charles "Tremendous" Jones, one of my great mentors, taught me it was okay to hug men. He hugged men in his church for years. Then he tried to quit, and the men would not let him. They were getting more hugging at church than they were getting at home all week.

Take care of yourself

Develop good habits

To live a long life, develop good health habits now. Don't smoke. Don't drink alcoholic beverages. Brush your teeth after every meal with a vibrating toothbrush.

My wife and I have traveled a great deal. We've never gotten sick during any of our travels. We've never been vaccinated before going abroad. We wash our hands often. We don't touch railings. We drink bottled water, watch where we eat, and don't get too much sun. We usually travel with another chiropractor so we have someone to treat us in the event we come down with some illness or injury.

Some of our missionary trips have been to very unhealthy areas. We take a lot of vitamins before our travels to build up our immunity.

When using public rest rooms I always put the towels down before washing my hands and after using the towels I open the door with the towels. Many people do not wash their hands after using the bathroom. Ugh!

All my smoking friends are dead

My father had his first heart attack at age 51. His second and fatal attack came just six years later. He began smoking in grade school. His two pack-a-day habit continued until his demise.

I can remember being sent to the store for cigarettes when we barely had food to eat. He didn't live long enough to know his grandchildren well.

My mother died at 28. Although her death was attributed to pneumonia, I believe it was from second-hand smoke and having six children in eight years.

My stepmother died several years ago. Smoking was never going to get her. After they found a spot on her lung and removed it, she died a horrible death losing eighty pounds the last year of her life.

When I began my chiropractic practice in Primghar, Iowa, in 1953 several of my colleagues in Northwest Iowa were smoking one to two packs a day. They're all dead now. Many of my former patients that I failed to convince to quit smoking are also dead.

My wife used to belong to a bridge club in Primghar. I wouldn't learn to play bridge because most of the players smoked. I couldn't stand the smoking environment. All the players who continued to smoke are dead, all from smoking related diseases. The non-smokers and those who quit are still alive.

Many of those people who died were encouraged to smoke by clever cigarette advertising that told them how wonderful and healthy smoking was for you. Doctors with stethoscopes around their necks told gullible audiences that smoking was good for your nerves and your health.

The ads also said that more doctors smoked their brand of cigarettes than any other brand. This was partly true. A week before the survey doctors got a free carton of cigarettes from that company. The people who said they'd walk a mile for a Camel cigarette can no longer walk anywhere.

The funniest show on television used to be "The Lucy and Desi Show." I'm still enjoying the reruns. Lucy and Desi are not. They both died from smoking related illnesses. Phillip Morris sponsored their show.

Remember "The Marlboro Man"? He was pictured riding horseback in the pristine mountain air. He died of cancer gasping for air. Remember Yul Brunner from "The King and I" fame? He was a three pack-a-day smoker who pleaded with people to quit smoking before his death from lung cancer. Remember how John Wayne died? Cancer of the lungs. Tough guy Steve McQueen could lick anything except cancer of the lungs. He died in his forties. They still show his greatest acting job on TV, "The Great Escape." He couldn't escape death from smoking cigarettes.

People are pictured in Washington marching on our legislators to outlaw guns. Five hundred times as many people die from smoking as from gun accidents and incidents.

Where are the marchers?

Smoking is an expensive and terrible health hazard. According to newspaper reports, it costs us taxpayers three dollars in health care costs and missed work for every pack of cigarettes smoked. Waitresses that work in restaurants that permit smoking have four times the incidence of lung cancer and two and one-half times the incidence of heart disease as unexposed waitresses do.

> **Worth a grin...**
>
> What's the difference between a nurse and a nun?
>
> A nun only serves one God.

Not a single person has died as a result of the smoking ban on the airlines or in California restaurants. Thousands of lives have been saved an extended as a result of those proscriptions.

Would you take a million dollars to quit? That's what it costs if you smoke from age 18 to age 65.

Young people today are encouraged to smoke because it looks "cool." It doesn't look "cool;" it looks dumb. Anyone who purposely puts health and welfare at risk doesn't look cool.

Our city, state, and national legislators should enact laws that protect the health and welfare of their constituents by restricting smoking in public places and work places that put non-smokers at risk.

When I began my practice in 1953 my colleagues told me I'd have to allow smoking in my office. I never did. Thousands of health-minded patients have thanked me for it. In the fifties I made up a sign for my office entitled "THANK YOU FOR NOT SMOKING." I got the idea from Braniff Airlines, which always thanked me for calling Braniff when I made reservations on their airline.

For years smokers were assured that smoking made them more alert, helped increase their concentration, and protected them against various forms of dementia and Alzheimer's Disease. Now we know better. Studies released in October of 2005 state that people who smoke have a diminished intelligence. Researchers found that older smokers were up to four times more likely to have evidence of significant intellectual decline than were persons who had never smoked or had quit smoking. The study took into account other factors that affect brain function among older persons, including depression and alcohol use.

So many friends who smoked are dead. Those who didn't die suffer from smoking-related diseases. Any way you look at it, smoking isn't worth it.

Bones and soda

Another disease problem is thinning bones or osteoporosis. Americans take more calcium and drink more milk than any other nation in the world and yet we have more women diagnosed with osteoporosis.

The reason is simple. We drink more soda drinks laced with phosphates that rob the body of calcium. Soda drinks are also high in sugar and caffeine, both of which deplete our bodies of calcium. We are constantly told by doctors to stay out of the sun, an excellent source of vitamin D, and we lack exercise that the rest of the world enjoys walking to work, bicycling, and not watching TV an average of seven hours each day.

Calcium tablets aren't sufficient to strengthen the bones because calcium requires many other nutrients to be absorbed properly. These include magnesium, phosphorous, vitamins A, K, D, and C, hydrochloric acid in the stomach, adequate protein and fat, iron, B_{12}, boron, manganese, and taurine.

Lift properly

Many industrial injuries and permanent injuries are the result of improper lifting. Always keep your spine perpendicular to the floor when lifting. Lift with your legs rather than your back. Keep your nose between your toes.

More spinal injuries occur in taller people, especially those taller than five feet, eight inches. According to the Harvard School of Medicine, fifty percent of people forty years or older have slipped, ruptured, or herniated discs. The U.S. government did a research project on back problems in 1994. They reported that only one percent of the patients having back surgery derived benefit from this dangerous procedure. Back surgery has also been reported to having caused fifty percent of the male candidates to become impotent.

Big breakfast

Breakfast is the most important meal of the day. You should eat your breakfast like a king, lunch like a prince and dinner like a pauper. Eating late in the evening will cause a tendency to over-eat. The consequences may be that you will push your blood sugar levels way up and have trouble sleeping.

Take a hot bath every day

I've learned that a hot bath can lower your blood pressure by as much as twenty millimeters of mercury. The reason is that hot baths dilate your blood vessels, and this lowers the blood pressure. Some people have the misconception that taking a hot bath raises blood pressure. It does increase the heart rate but does not normally raise blood pressure. Taking a hot bath just before retiring helps you fall into a deep, untroubled sleep. I do not recommend more than half an hour in a bathtub.

Keep the same daily schedule

I have found that patients usually have headaches on Sunday. This is because on Sunday they change their routine.

Your body becomes accustomed to rising and retiring at the same hour. I tell people who don't work on week ends to get up at the same hour, eat the same breakfast, and take a brisk walk before getting involved in physical and mental activities throughout the day. Too many men suffer from backache on Sunday from sitting in a recliner watching football games on TV.

I do not recommend recliners for people with bad backs. Every time they lean back in the chair, they crunch down on their discs. Sitting in the recliner four or five hours watching TV is not a healthy activity. You would be much better served playing touch football with your children or grandchildren—or the kids up the street.

Vitamins and minerals

Many doctors tell their patients not to worry about vitamins and minerals because they get all they need from the foods they eat.

Nothing could be farther from the truth. Only the most ideal circumstances would allow a person to eat a perfect diet with all the nutrients needed for good health. A survey of the eating habits of 15,000 people a few years ago by Dr. Emanuel Cheraskin, author of *Predictive Medicine*, found that eighty-five percent were deficient in one or more nutrients, and the majority were deficient in several.

The problem is that most of our foods are grown in soil that has been depleted of its original mineral content. Farmers today add only nitrogen, phosphorous, and potash to the depleted soil. Organic fertilizers are added only rarely, and the topsoil continues to erode.

At my free health clinics in Jamaica, Poland, and the Ukraine, I was amazed by the health and physical well being of those patients compared to our typical American patient. Most of our foreign patients, I learned, walked to work, had big gardens, caught fresh fish out of the ocean, didn't watch TV seven hours a day, didn't sit in a Lazy Boy recliner and didn't take a handful of pills at every meal. Many have never seen a doctor, and they weren't trying to keep up with the Joneses. In Jamaica they expressed their calmness by saying, "Jamaica, no problem, man."

Most of us Americans have no idea about the adverse effects our daily habits have on the absorption, assimilation, and utilization of the nutrients we ingest. For example, if you smoke, you are losing vitamins A, D, B_1, B_2, B_3, B_5, B_6, B_{12}, C, the bioflavinoids, biotin, and folic acid. See Appendix page 180 for a list of common vitamin and mineral deficiencies caused by various substances.

The value of vitamins

Five medical doctors on a Sioux Falls television interview program were asked if there are any vitamins that help prevent or cure cancer. They all agreed that they didn't know of any nutrients that would do that. They were wrong. There are several vitamins that help prevent cancer: A, C, E, selenium, zinc, and calcium. Several articles have appeared in the national news about calcium preventing bowel cancer.

I believe I have a full head of hair into my seventies because I take a lot of the right kind of vitamins. Good nutrition has also helped me go to work without missing one day for fifty years.

> Not long ago, dog food companies were spending more money on nutritional research for dogs than scientists were spending studying human nutrition.

The reason most physicians lack nutrition information is that while medicines can be patented and sold for fantastic profits, nutrients cannot. It's as simple as that. It doesn't make economic sense to direct research towards the nutritional treatment of disease. A few years ago dog food companies were spending more money on nutritional research for dogs than scientists were spending on human nutrition.

Two out of three adult Americans take some form of vitamins and minerals to supplement their diet. It is my professional opinion that everyone ought to be taking vitamin and mineral supplements. One reason is that for every dollar spent on nutritional supplements, several dollars are saved in health care expenses. Doesn't it make sense to nourish the organs and tissues of your body without medication or surgery? You need good nutrition from the cradle to the grave.

It is rare that I find a patient who is eating a well-balanced, all-inclusive, nutritional diet. Even if you are eating healthy foods but are also taking soda pop, antacids, caffeine, birth control pills, alcohol, or tobacco, enduring stress, or sweating profusely, you will lose essential nutrients from your body.

It is amusing to me that minimal daily requirements are set up without regard to the weight or lifestyle of the individual. An adult 85-pound woman has the same daily requirements for essential nutrients as does the 400-pound woman. A patient who is deficient in iron may test high in iron levels the next day after a dinner of liver.

Many food products we eat were harvested months or even years before and have been in storage. This deteriorates the vitamin and mineral content. I once read a comment in a farm magazine that an apple orchard had been sprayed thirty-two times before the apples were harvested.

Archeologists have found evidence in skeletons preserved by favorable weather conditions indicating that people who ate food from trees, gardens, and plants had stronger teeth and spines than those who utilized the typical Western diet.

Vitamin C

A Harvard study in Finland found that mega doses of Vitamin C, more than 700 milligrams per day over a ten-year period, can reduce risk of heart disease by 25 percent. In the middle of the twentieth century the recommended daily allowance for Vitamin C was ten milligrams. It was raised later to 95 milligrams per day, a 950 percent increase in fifty years. Many nutritionists believe it should be closer to 500 milligrams per day. Man is one of only three animal species that do not store Vitamin C in their bodies. That means we have to replenish the vitamin every day.

Vitamin therapy

The Physicians' Desk Reference (PDR) reported last year that 65 percent of our senior population is now taking vitamins. That's good news. Vitamins offer protection and cures for many common ailments.

If you take aspirin, antibiotics, estrogen or cholesterol drugs; drink alcohol and caffeine drinks, use birth control pills, eat sugar, smoke cigarettes, and sweat a lot, you may be vitamin and mineral deficient.

Be careful what you buy and use. The cheapest vitamins are usually the most expensive. Natural vitamin E is made from soybeans. Cheap vitamin E is made from petroleum. Which do you suppose is better for you? Health food store vitamins are usually made from natural products.

Chiropractors and naturopaths are both well trained in vitamin therapies and many times have vitamins available for their patients. Medical doctors are not well trained in nutrition. Their training is mainly supported by drug companies. Vitamins are natural substances and cannot be patented.

The common cold

The common cold costs us $40 billion a year. Absenteeism from work and school and the effects of medication are responsible for most of these costs.

In any given year, three out of four Americans will have two or more colds. It is the most common human illness. Respiratory infections and allergies account for eighty percent of all doctor office visits.

Antibiotics have no effect on the common cold, but 41 million prescriptions for antibiotics are written each year to treat people with a cold. One result of overprescribing antibiotics is the development of resistance by antibiotics to specific strains of viruses.

Most cold sufferers will get better on their own without a visit to the doctor. In fact, the doctor's office is a good place to catch a cold.

The best way to avoid colds is to stay home, drink plenty of fluid, and get seven to nine hours of sleep each day. Research has shown that vitamin A and C and the mineral zinc help shorten the length of a cold.

Don't shake hands with people who are coughing, sneezing, or blowing their noses. Remember that sugar attacks your natural immunity by reducing your white blood count. Leave it alone.

The benefits of massage therapy

As I've mentioned elsewhere in this book, we have four massage therapists at our clinic. We believe that the therapy these talented care givers provide is a major factor in the return to health of our patients.

Some people think that massage therapy is primarily useful in helping a person relax tense and sore muscles. Much more than that is going on. A stressful encounter causes a nervous reaction that triggers a flight-or-fight response involving our sympathetic nervous system. Our muscles tighten, our hair stands on end, and we breathe more rapidly.

After danger has passed, the other part of our Autonomic Nervous System (ANS), the parasympathetic nervous system, is activated. Your body relaxes, and your heart rate, breathing, and blood flow to your muscles all slow down so that your body can resume its normal state of relaxation—until the next stressful event occurs.

If you load too much stress, your body becomes filled with toxins, and you can become ill. Many people suffer from stress-related diseases, and massage is an excellent way to bring your parasympathetic nervous system into an active state so that you can enjoy an alert and relaxed state of awareness.

Laura Sadler, a certified massage therapist, Reiki Master, and Yoga instructor in Los Angeles, describes specific health benefits of massage like this:

> Toxins are eliminated through the movement of blood and lymph during the massage. Although the blood flow to the muscles slows during a massage, while the therapist is working on a specific muscle, blood flow is increased in the area of contact, and ultimately circulation does increase in the body after a massage. When blood circulation increases, it increases the oxygen to the cells and thus increases elimination of toxins...

> Another benefit of massage is that it can relieve chronic pain or muscle tension. A weekly massage can help to retrain the muscles to relax. Our nerves and muscles have memory. When we experience stress or trauma even though we may not think about it after a while, our nerves and muscles will remember the experience. This can often lead to muscles staying contracted or in spasm in an effort to guard the body against the stress or trauma...

> Just by taking the time to enjoy a relaxing therapeutic massage, you are truly allowing your body to rejuvenate and detoxify. In the environment that we live and work in, anything that we can do to improve our health will help our body to serve us better and longer.

Use your head and save your back

Eighty-five percent of all Americans will have a problem with their back sometime during their life.

The importance of chiropractic care

The adult spine is composed of 26 movable bones or verte-brae. The most important function of your spine is to house and protect your nervous system.

The brain communicates with your body systems, organs, and tissues, controlling all body functions either directly or indi-rectly. It is therefore imperative that your spine be free of mis-alignments. A pinched nerve can cause disease. Chiropractors are especially trained to locate and correct spinal misalignments with the use of X-ray, instrumentation, muscle testing, and physical findings.

Here's how you can prevent a visit to a chiropractor by using your head to save your back. When lifting, hold the load close to your body. Bend your knees and not your back. Don't jump off platforms, hay racks, and out of tractor cabs. Don't lift and twist at the same time. Change your posture frequently at work. Avoid sitting for over an hour at a time. Get out of your car at least once an hour. Allow plenty of time in your travels. Women should not carry purses over their shoulder and shouldn't load them down with surplus items.

Football collisions and car crashes frequently result in severe spinal problems. Use handrails on steps and use night lights to prevent falling in the dark. Don't leave items on the floor or walkways that you might trip over in your traffic pattern at home or at work.

Avoid unnecessary travel or walking on ice. If you fall and break a hip there's a twenty-five percent chance you won't sur-vive a year. Avoid drugs that cause dizziness. If you drink alcohol drink in moderation. Many car accidents and bad falls happen to people under the influence.

The four most dangerous jobs for back injuries are handling heavy materials, driving trucks, working as a nurse, and farming.

The Harvard School of Medicine reported several years ago that half of all people over forty years of age have slipped, rup-tured, or herniated discs. Most disc problems occur from a severe wrenching of the spine or lifting too heavy an object.

Can chiropractors treat a slipped disc without surgery? Absolutely! The only reason a disc becomes displaced is from the vertebrae being twisted, squeezing the disc and pushing it against nerves. That's why your arms, hands, or legs ache and go numb. Chiropractic adjustments can alleviate the pain and discomfort of a slipped disc. What about surgery? In 1994 a report showed that only one person in one hundred is helped by back surgery for any reason, including a slipped disc.

Irregularity

There is little that will help your health more than regular bowel movements. You should experience one to three bowel movements daily unless you eat very little food.

Most cases of constipation can be cured by chiropractic adjustments. The nerves lead to the bowels and cause peristaltic action to take place. Remember that laxatives don't move the bowels; the bowels move the laxative. Laxatives are powerful irritants that cause the bowels to contract to get rid of the poison and as a result the bowels move. Continued use of laxatives cause great damage to the intestinal tract. One of the chemicals utilized in laxatives is stronger than lye. If you take it when you have appendicitis, it will cause your appendix to rupture.

It is easy to help people with constipation. First, they should drink more water, half an ounce for every pound of body weight, more if you are working in a hot environment or if you participate in strenuous physical activity. A second remedy is magnesium tablets, which will help eliminate constipation. Third, fruits and vegetables and high fiber diets all are of great benefit to irregular patients. Finally, eat a few prunes or figs before you go to bed at night or early in the morning.

Just because the label says it is natural doesn't prove that it is.

Many people develop constipation by refusing to heed the symptoms of a bowel movement. They work in a job where they cannot conveniently take off and use the restroom. As a result of holding back they develop chronic constipation.

Nothing concerns a mother or grandmother more than constipation. I have found that about eighty percent of my patients suffer from constipation. Articles in health columns by medical experts say it's all right if you have a bowel movement only once a week. Nonsense. Good health demands that the bowels move once or twice each day. Fecal matter is waste matter and is toxic if not eliminated in a timely manner.

I have no problems eliminating my patient's constipation problems. You need an optimal nerve supply to the large intestine (colon) and rectum. If your feces float in the water it means you have enough fiber in your diet. Eating prunes and prune juice activates the bowel. Drinking warm water upon retiring and arising is often helpful. I recommend dietary fiber tablets that contain psyllium seed, citrus pectin, agar, and guar gum.

Drink more water. Take magnesium tablets and increase your vitamin C levels.

Many drugs cause constipation problems. Check to see if that is a possible side effect and if it is, talk to your doctor about eliminating it.

Harsh laxatives should never be taken, especially if you have pain in the lower right quadrant of the abdomen. Harsh laxatives could rupture your appendix. When you have the urge to defecate, go; otherwise you may develop chronic constipation problems.

Constipation and diarrhea

Eighty percent of the adult population in the United States have bowel problems. Eighty percent of this eighty percent have constipation problems and the other twenty percent have problems with diarrhea. Normal bowel activity is essential for good health. You can help maintain normal bowel activity by drinking normal amounts of water (eight to ten glasses per day), the ingestion of adequate bulk mainly from fruits and vegetables and whole grain cereals. It is also essential to exercise by walking, swimming or biking.

Another essential activity that will help bowel function is taking the time to go to the bathroom. The most important factor in bowel activity is a normal nerve supply from the brain, through the spine and the intestinal tract. The nerves control the major functions of both the small and the large intestine. Nerves maintain the activity of peristalsis, the process of the bowel contracting and moving the waste material along until it is eventually eliminated by defecation.

Personal appearance

Well dressed people with good personal hygiene respond better than poorly dressed patients with poor personal hygiene. Did you hear about the guy who had bad breath? He spent thousands of dollars to get rid of his problem but found out people still didn't like being around him. He got rid of his problem by going to a psychiatrist.

You might ask, "How can a psychiatrist help bad breath?" The answer is, they can't, but now the guy with bad breath doesn't give a damn about it.

Don't carry your purse over your shoulder

A woman carrying her purse over her shoulder usually elevates her shoulder to keep her purse from falling off. Therein lies the problem. Carrying a purse like this puts extra strain on the neck and thoracic vertebrae.

A solution would be to remove all excess items so that you don't have to carry a bowling ball in the opposite hand to balance your spine.

Good health, naturally

Water

The earth and our bodies are made up of approximately seventy percent water. I wonder if that is one of God's plans.

Almost every recommendation for the consumption of water each day has been to drink eight glasses each day. My sister-in-law weighs 85 pounds and one of my sons weighs 325. Do they both need eight glasses each day?

Assuredly not. The proper prescription for water each day is one-half ounce per pound of body weight. This can also vary if you sweat a lot, are taking diuretic drugs, are diabetic, use caffeine, are flying at a high altitude, are under stress, are undergoing radiation therapy, or are engaged in excessive physical activity.

I do not recommend fluoridated or chlorinated water because both of these chemicals are extremely toxic, even in small dosages. I have a filter in my refrigerator but it does not remove fluoride from the water. I do not recommend distilled water because some essential minerals are lacking.

Bottled water is usually in a bottle made from petroleum, which may be toxic. There is a plant in Blair, Nebraska, that is making bottles from corn. I certainly hope they will soon be providing drinking water in those bottles.

They make filters now that you can put on your shower head or bathtub head to remove chemicals from the water you bathe in. Treated water even in small dosages can adversely affect your health.

If you have access to a spring or artesian well and the water has been tested for safety, go for it. Half the water in the U.S. has some safety factor problems.

Fluorine is odorless, colorless, and tasteless. The fluoride found in soils is far different than the toxic chemical they add in fluoridation of city water supplies. Fluoride is needed in the first eight years of life for normal dentition. After that, the use of fluoridated toothpaste, fluorine in vitamins, and too much in your water supply could wreak havoc with your health.

We have a carbon water filter on our refrigerator. It improves most of the impurities and bad taste but does not remove fluoride. The only way to remove fluoride is to use a distiller, but then you lose all of the minerals. Most filtered water comes in plastic bottles made out of petroleum products. Fortunately there is now a new process where they are making bottles out of corn. This should be less intrusive on our health.

Many health problems respond well to the increased consumption of water.

The air you breathe

The quality of your health depends a great deal upon the air you breathe. A few generations ago doctors were encouraging us to smoke cigarettes because it was supposed to relax your nerves and soothe your throat. After years of polluting smokers' lungs, a whole army of lung cancer patients was created.

You don't have to smoke to breathe the polluted air of those who do smoke. Non-smokers at cocktail parties have been shown to have seventy percent of the level of nicotine that their smoking party-goers had. Secondhand smoke has also been implicated for causing cancer of the breast.

It behooves us to breathe the healthiest air possible. Here are some suggestions:

- Use a good furnace filter.

- Live in an area that has lots of trees because they take in carbon dioxide and convert it to oxygen.

- Air out your house, especially after a rain storm.

- Sleep with your bedroom window open.

- Avoid working in a polluted area and along busy streets with several lanes of traffic.

- Choose a job that does not require you to breathe in exhaust gases, welding by-products, insecticides and pesticides.

- Use the carbon filter on late model cars when traveling in heavy traffic, through smoke, or blowing dirt or sand.

- Do not permit people to smoke in your house or work place.

- If you smoke, quit. If you don't smoke, don't start.

Sunshine and fresh air

We need more sunshine. I'm not advocating sunburn, but sunshine is good for you. Hypocrites, the father of modern medicine, recommended sunshine and fresh air as important in gaining and maintaining good health. One of the great injustices of modern medicine is cautioning patients to stay out of the sun. Submariners during World War II suffered from major illnesses due to the lack of sunshine.

Sunshine activates several important biological functions within the human body. Sunshine converts the 7-dehydrocholesterol on your skin to vitamin D, which is anticarcinogenic against breast and colon cancer. The 7-dehydrocholesterol on the skin transformed into vitamin D helps to build strong bones and teeth. Sunshine also activates the hypothalamus, parathyroid, pineal and pituitary glands into performing such important functions as energy, appetite, body temperature, sleep and the balance of fluids in the body.

Howard Warp, the founder of Pioneer Village, in Minden, Nebraska, discovered that chickens laid more eggs when the windows of chicken houses were covered with plastic rather than glass because glass filters out UV radiation.

Years ago everyone who wore glasses had heavy glass lenses that filtered out UV light. When exposed to the sun they all looked like owls. Their faces were tanned but their eyes were white.

Naturally I advise patients to avoid getting a sunburn. However, I encourage them to get as much sunlight as possible. I also recommend that they wear glasses that allow natural sunlight into the eyes.

Do you realize that we have far more skin cancers in the northern part of the United States than in the southern sunshine states? Australia is a nation of sun worshippers but they have fewer incidences of skin cancers than we do.

Farmers learned a long time ago that livestock raised in confinement have a host of health problems due to the lack of sunshine.

Sleep

A good night's sleep is essential to good health and longevity. You should have seven to nine hours of sound sleep every night. Unfortunately, that's the exception and not the norm. If you sleep less than seven hours you are not charging your batteries. If you require more than nine hours you probably have some health issues. One third of our adult population suffers from insomnia.

There are many things that you can do to afford yourself the luxury of good sleep habits, for example:

1. Go to bed and arise at the same time each day.

2. Don't drink anything with caffeine in it after 3 p.m.

3. Don't watch horror stories before retiring.

4. Sleep in a darkened room with fresh air at a comfortable temperature.

5. Sleep on a good sleep product preferably with a cotton top and cotton sheets.

6. Take a warm bath or Jacuzzi before retiring.

7. Don't sleep on your stomach. It puts a bad kink in your neck.

8. Keep your spine in line. If you sleep on your side use two pillows, one under your head and the other between your knees.

9. Think positive thoughts before retiring.

10. Be thankful for all the good things in your life.

11. Avoid drugs that excite you and sleeping pills that may become habit forming. One to three milligrams of melatonin may be a helpful sleep aid but don't let it become a habit.

12. Say your prayers and read your Bible

13. Don't have a clock or a telephone near your head.

14. Play soft melodious music.

15. Watch something humorous before retiring.

16. Certain vitamins and minerals have a calming effect upon the body. Vitamin C, calcium, magnesium, and potassium have a calming effect.

17. Chamomile tea helps many of my patients get a better night's sleep.

18. Don't eat a heavy meal late at night just before retiring.

19. Sleep in a quiet room.

20. Remove watches and other jewelry before retiring.

A good mattress is hard to find but is essential in obtaining a good night's sleep. When you find a mattress you think will be right for you, don't purchase it without a warranty. You may want to take it back later.

I have not found water beds to be a benefit to myself or my patients. My wife complained from day one when we had a water bed. I do not believe that the water causes the problem but that the electrical heating coils and the plastic that contains the water are the factors that cause trouble.

Natural nutrition

A degree in medicine includes minimal instruction in nutrition in its effect on the health and well-being of patients. Dr. Emanuel Cheraskin, a doctor who does know a lot about nutritional therapy, said, "The average medical doctor knows a little more about nutrition than his secretary, unless his secretary has a weight problem. Then she knows more than he does." Cheraskin is the author of many fine books on nutrition including *Predictive Medicine.*

As one who has studied nutrition for more than fifty years, I have come to the conclusion that most diseases of mankind have a nutritional component. As a consequence, many of the major diseases of mankind can be helped by a proper diet and by proper intake of vitamins and minerals, enzymes, and herbs.

While we were living and practicing in Sioux Center, Iowa, my wife told me that the local medical doctor was going to give a lecture on nutrition at the women's club. When he got up to speak, it became apparent that most of the women knew more about nutrition than he did. He confessed that his entire study of nutrition took place in one afternoon in medical school.

Many medical doctors today are learning more and more about natural products and natural treatment protocols. They are recommending magnesium for high blood pressure as well as calcium. They are recommending herbs for the reduction of cholesterol.

A book, *Prescription for Nutritional Healing,* by James F. Balch, M.D., a doctor who practices medicine in the specialty of urology, includes detailed explanations of what natural products you might take and what natural things you might utilize to recover from most of the diseases of mankind.

Eat organic foods

Foods grown organically are much more available now than they used to be. Most supermarkets, health food stores, farmers' markets, and flea markets have organic products available. Organic foods are raised on soils that were not commercially fertilized, and no insecticides or herbicides were used in growing or processing the food products. Meat products of animals raised either on grass or grains without the ingestion of drugs, vaccinations, or hormones are available at certain meat processing lockers or plants.

Your environment

Where you live and where you work may have a great effect on your longevity. I think the best place to live and work would be to on a lake in Minnesota in the summer time and in Hawaii in the winter. Sunshine and fresh air are good for a person.

I practiced in two rural communities in Iowa for thirty-eight years. There was little pollution by traffic and we had a lot of trees in those communities. Trees take in carbon dioxide and give back oxygen. You're better off to live in an area with lots of sunshine and fresh air.

My home is in a secluded area with very little traffic and lots of trees. My office, unfortunately, is in a very heavily traveled area with seven lanes on one side of our building and four lanes on the other side. Since practicing in the heavily traveled area my yearly hair analysis has shown a marked increase in cadmium, an industrial pollutant.

Keep chemicals out of drinking water

The manufacturing of 200,000 airplanes made primarily of aluminum helped us win World War II. One of the by-products of the production of aluminum was thousands of tons of aluminum fluoride, a very toxic poison. When released into our streams it caused great problems of pollution. Fluoride is used as an insecticide to kill rodents, cockroaches, and lice. It also has a mild benefit in the first five years of life in the development of normal teeth.

At the beginning of the twentieth century it was discovered that residents of Texas and Colorado had dental fluorosis (mottled teeth) and that the children with fluorosis had fewer cavities. The source of the fluoride was calcium fluoride, a natural mineral. Since 1980 sodium hexafluorosilicate and hexafluorosilicate acid have been substituted for naturally occurring calcium fluoride. Studies in the past fifteen years show only slight benefits for children from three to five years of age.

Harmful side effects of fluoridation include tooth and bone fractures and increased cancer rates.

An Alcoa chemist conducted a fluoridation experiment on rats and reported that fluoridation of water reduced cavities in rats. (Frankly, I've never seen a rat with cavities.) After that several industries got together using flawed epidemiology studies that have now been discredited, and proposed that the nation's water supplies be fluoridated at 1 part per million.

Experiments were conducted for a ten-year period in three cities: Evanston, Illinois; Newburgh, New York; and Grand Rapids, Michigan. After five years the experiments were halted because researchers claimed the evidence showed that cavities had been reduced by two-thirds. Is five years long enough to evaluate complications of such a toxic chemical? Fluoridated water is not recommended for children under three or over five or for adults.

According to Dr. Robert Mendelson, "the people's doctor," all three of the towns where the experiments took place in the late 1940s now have three times as many dentists per 10,000 residents as in prefluoridation times.

You have to wonder how much sense it makes to conclude that dental caries declined by two-thirds over a five-year period when tests showed that fluoridation helps children only slightly during a three-year span.

An interesting side note concerns Oscar Ewing, who as the Assistant Director of the Democratic Party worked to discredit Vice President Henry Wallace and win the election of Harry Truman as Vice President. Later, after Truman became President, he rewarded Ewing by naming him Director of the Federal Security Administration. Since Alcoa was one of the greatest producers of aluminum fluoride, it was only natural that every medical doctor and dentist was soon bombarded with favorable information. Fluoridation of water was heavily promoted by the Federal Security Administration, which later became the Department of Health, Education, and Welfare.

The "father of public relations," Edward L. Bernays, handled much of the promotion of fluoridation. He knew how to influence opinion by his work with the tobacco companies to convince women to take up smoking. This was during the days in 1950s when we saw television advertising with doctors telling us that smoking calms the nervous and soothes throats.

The current method of manufacturing fluoride leaves residues of toxic metals such as lead, arsenic, cadmium, and mercury. Austria, Denmark, Finland, France, Italy, Belgium, Switzerland, Luxemburg, Norway, Spain, Greece, Japan, Hungary, Portugal, and Germany no longer subscribe for fluoridation.

Dr. H. Trendley Dean, head of the Dental Hygiene Unit at the National Institute of Health (NIH), began investigating the epidemiology of fluorosis in 1931. He has twice confessed in court that earlier studies he relied on were invalid. A study in 1955 found that children aged 7-14 in Kingston, New York, an unfluoridated town, had less tooth decay and half as much mottling as those in Newburgh. The studies were conducted by the New York Health Department.

An Iowa dentist went to the town council and asked them to fluoridate the water because of all the tooth decay in his town. When they examined the water they found it had too much fluoride.

Dental experts advise that children under three should not use fluoridated toothpaste and that babies should never have their formula mixed with water that contains fluorine. Vancouver, Canada, which does not have fluoridation, has a lower cavity rate than does Toronto, which does fluoridate.

After twenty years of fluoridation, ten of the largest fluoridated cities have seen a ten percent increase in cancer compared with rates in nonfluoridated cities. In Utah hip fractures are double in 75-year-old women who live in fluoridated cities compared to women of the same age in nonfluoridated cities. Gerald F. Judd, Ph.D., has listed 113 ailments caused by fluorine in our bodies.

I could go on with more pages of severe and unpredictable health problems, but space does not permit me to do so. My biggest concern relates to terrorism in the world today. What would happen if terrorists broke into our water processing plants and released excessive amounts of fluorine into our drinking water? Fluorine is colorless, odorless, and tasteless. The fluoride ions are so small they would pass right through our finest filters. We could be poisoned before we know it.

The information in the above pages is from an article in the *Journal of Physicians and Surgeons,* Vol. 10, No. 3, Summer 2005, by Joel M. Kauffman, Ph.D., Professor of Chemistry Emeritus at the University of the Sciences in Philadelphia, Pennsylvania.

Sobriety

I'm a total abstainer. I've never been drunk in my life. My last drink was more than twenty-five years ago. My father was an alcoholic who managed to ruin the lives of all those around him. He finally sobered up for the last fifteen years of his life.

Alcoholism affects one out of every ten people. The costs of drinking are astronomical. The county sheriff told me years ago that nine out of ten of his prisoners were in jail because of alcohol. They drank and wrote a bad check, stole something, beat up their spouse and drove drunk. Many drivers today are going to jail for years for killing an innocent person. For many alcoholics one drink is too many, and 100 is not enough.

Alcohol destroys brain cells. Yes, I know that they have found out that a couple of glasses of red wine are good for your health. I discuss that in a section on page 141 entitled, "The French Paradox."

For those of you who tell me about all the wine mentioned in the Bible, let me remind you that the distillation of alcohol did not take place until 400 AD, so the liquor that was consumed in the Bible was probably little more than fermented grape juice.

Exercise

Don't jog on hard surfaces. The pressure on joints and ligaments from hard contact with a pavement or sidewalk can injure joint or tissues in the feet, ankles, knees, and hips. Grass, blacktop, and dirt surfaces are much better on your body.

Jogging is great for your health but can be dangerous if you quit suddenly and allow your muscular heart to build up with fat instead of muscle.

Walking is one of the cheapest means of daily exercise. You need to walk at least a mile at a time to do yourself a real health favor. Three is better than one. Golfing is a great way to get your three miles in—if you don't use a cart.

I don't recommend walking in a shopping mall unless they have carpeted floors.

Many cities now have scenic trails. You might also walk to work. I did for five years and lost forty pounds in the process.

Watch your posture when you walk. Stand straight and walk with your head held high. Get together with a friend to share the joy of walking.

I have made nearly a dozen trips to foreign countries providing free chiropractic clinics to the lost, the lame and the lonely. I've been amazed at how much faster and more complete the recoveries of my foreign patients have been compared to the outcomes of my American patients.

I'm certain the difference is due to the physical condition of our patients. My overseas patients walk several miles to get to work, don't sit in overstuffed furniture, and don't watch TV for an average of seven hours each day. They spend their evenings working in their gardens or yards and don't ride around in golf carts.

The very best exercise is swimming because you use all of your long muscles and oxygenate your lungs. Because swimming is not an option for many patients, the next best exercise is walking, followed by cycling, walking up stairs, gardening, raking, dancing, playing tennis, or walking the golf course. A rebounder (a miniature trampoline) is great for your legs and lungs. These three-foot devices are available for under fifty dollars.

Try walking or cycling to work. Walk up the stairs instead of using the elevator. Park your car as far from your work station as is possible. Take long walks with loved ones. Climb mountains or hills. Stay out of the malls for exercise unless they are carpeted.

Exercise should be performed daily by the diabetic and hypertensive patient.

My favorite is swimming. Walking or biking is usually more affordable and convenient. It's best to have a companion accompanying you to maintain your dedication. A minimum of thirty minutes must be performed to be of benefit.

A thirty-minute workout on a three-foot trampoline in front of the television is an inexpensive alternative.

Tennis, bicycling, badminton, table tennis, golf (if you stay out of the golf cart), handball and racquet ball are other excellent ways to enjoy good exercise.

It is my professional opinion that a sensible diet plus an hour of exercise a day—walking, swimming, or bicycling— would extend your life expectancy by several years and give you significantly lower risks of heart attack, stroke, degenerative disease, and dementia.

When I conduct free clinics for the people in Poland, I find them to be in much better health than U.S. citizens. I think much of this is due to the fact that they love their gardens. They spend their weekends working in their garden.

There is a two fold benefit from having a garden: You grow your own organic foods free of pesticides and herbicides and without commercial fertilizers; and fresh fruits and vegetables are much better for you than the produce bought in the super market. That produce may have been harvested more than a year ago, treated with chemicals and irradiation, stored under adverse conditions with the result that it is of little nutritive value to you. Maybe the passion for gardening is the reason you almost never see a golf course in Poland.

Wear proper footwear and orthotics

I've seen thousands of patients who are suffering with hammer toes, bunions, fallen arches, and heel spurs. Most of these problems are caused by poorly fitting shoes and cheap footwear.

Hammer toes and bunions are usually caused by wearing shoes that are too short. Heel spurs and fallen arches can be ameliorated by wearing shoe inserts that cradle the spur and support the arch. The best one I've used is made by Foot Levelers and can be obtained at www.FootLevelers.com. The best shoes I've ever worn are made by Allen Edmonds.

When your feet hurt you do hurt all over.

Cowboy boots are sometimes better than regular shoes. If your feet are comfortable, chances are you're wearing the right foot wear.

Natural remedies

There are natural remedies for most diseases. Kevin Trudeau has written a book, *Natural Cures They Don't Want You to Know About.* He has some excellent ideas on how to treat yourself naturally. Health food stores are great sources for foods and other items to aid in the natural treatment of many common illnesses.

The trend is toward the choice of alternative medical care, as reported by *USA Today* in June of 2004. The following percentages show that there is a strong preference for wholistic medicine over traditional medicine at all age levels:

Percentage preferring holistic medicine

Ages 18 to 34	18%
Ages 35 to 49	24%
Ages 50 to 64	23%
Ages 65+	15%

There are nutritional components to many diseases. Specific cures are available and sometimes it's possible to avoid disease by taking certain vitamins and minerals. Many medical doctors are switching from traditional medical procedures to alternative methods. The good news is that treatment with natural methods is many times more effective and at a much lower cost.

Dr. David Isenberg of the Harvard School of Medicine has reported that sick people are now visiting alternative practitioners more frequently than ordinary MDs. These practitioners include chiropractors, acupuncture practitioners, massage therapists, nutrition experts, and herbologists. Many patients have to pay out of their own pockets for this alternative treatment. Obviously it is of greater value to them than are insurance-covered services.

Proper driving habits

Many of the health problems of Americans have been caused by spinal and nervous system damage caused by vehicle crashes. Almost 50,000 people die each year on our highways and roads. Many victims of traffic crashes have their longevity compromised by "whiplash" accidents. Uncorrected spinal misalignments may cause pressure on intervertebral discs, the spinal cord, and the nerves as they pass between the vertebrae.

When I first began practicing fifty-two years ago we rarely saw victims of whiplash accidents with severe spinal damage showing on their X-rays. Today they are ubiquitous. Fifty years ago people drove an average of five thousand miles each year. Today it's more like fifty thousand miles each year. The speed limit was thirty-five miles an hour during World War II. Today it's seventy-five on our super highways. Drivers aren't nearly as courteous today. You've heard of "road rage," I'm sure.

During my sixty years of driving I've never caused an accident. Some rules for avoiding accidents and subsequent injuries are as follow:

1. Leave early and allow adequate time for travel.

2. Practice defensive and courteous driving.

3. Look both ways twice before entering an intersection.

4. Avoid medications that may impair your judgment.

5. Avoid drinking and driving.

6. Get out of your car every hour and stretch (Rest stops are about seventy miles apart on the Interstate.)

7. Never drive when tired.

8. Don't follow too closely.

9. Buckle up. It's the law in most states.

10. Make certain your brakes work.

Deficiencies and hair

Several years ago Dr. William Risley informed me about the benefits of hair analysis. Having worked my way through high school on farms I was well aware of the fact that many farmers could tell an animal was sick by examining their hair coat. I collected hair samples of two of my problem patients and sent them in for an analysis without informing them of the symptoms of my patients. The analysis came back with the exact symptomatology of both patients.

One of my patients had an irregular heart for more than thirty years. A hair sample found him deficient in copper. After prescribing copper for the patient his irregular heartbeat disappeared.

Blood samples may be normal if you ate certain foods the night before. Hair analysis is more likely to show chronic deficiencies or excessive levels of minerals or toxic metals. Dr. Risley's analysis also includes recommended dietary changes and nutritional supplementation to correct abnormal levels of your body chemistry. For further information about hair analysis, you can call Dr. Risley, Analytical Labs, 602 995-1580.

Here is a list of vitamins and minerals you need for healthy hair, and the way a deficiency of these nutrients may be apparent in your hair.

Vitamins

Vitamin A: Dry, brittle hair

Vitamin E: Dull, dry hair

Vitamin F: Lusterless and brittle hair

Vitamin B_5 (pantothenic acid): hair turns gray

Vitamin C: loss of hair

Biotin: baldness

Choline: baldness

Inositol: baldness

PABA: gray hair

Minerals

Chloride: loss of hair

Copper: loss of hair color

Iodine: dry hair

Iron: loss of hair

Selenium: dandruff

Another Essential Nutrient

Protein: loss of hair

112 ideas that may help you live to be 100

Eat better

1. Follow a healthy diet

2. Avoid sugar, salt, and white flour

3. Take vitamins

4. Drink plenty of water

5. Eat organic foods

6. Avoid food additives

7. Control your weight

8. Believe in the French Paradox

9. Avoid trans-fatty acids

10. Don't eat fast foods

11. Remember that if it's advertised on TV it's probably not good for you

12. Don't microwave your food

13. Avoid food in aluminum cans and aluminum cookware

14. Avoid artificial sweeteners

15. Eat several small meals

16. Always eat a big breakfast

17. Keep from eating white bread. The whiter the bread the quicker you're dead.

18. Plant a garden and grow your own food

Take care of yourself

19. Exercise at least thirty minutes every day

20. Get some sunshine when you can

21. Sleep well

22. Choose chiropractic care

23. Respect your environment

24. Try to live in a healthy location

25. Pick healthy ancestors

26. Stay sober

27. Encourage your own healthful personal habits

28. Avoid OTC and prescription drugs

29. Take good care of your personal appearance

30. Use cosmetics with care

31. Choose comfortable clothing

32. Promote regularity

33. Prefer natural remedies

34. Avoid EMFs (electro-magnetic fields)

35. Try to breathe healthy air

36. Minimize the use of cell phones

37. Stay out of the way of TV radiation

38. Avoid sprays around the house

39. Avoid fluoridation and fluoride supplemented products

40. Choose a car with solid safety features

41. Don't "Super size" anything

42. Avoid non-stick cookware

43. Don't use deodorants made with aluminum

44. Avoid sitting for long hours

45. Develop proper sleeping habits

46. Follow proper driving habits

47. Wear proper footwear and orthotics

48. Don't wear your purse over your shoulder.

49. Don't use fluorescent lights

50. Don't jog on hard surfaces

51. Sell your motorcycle, or at least wear a helmet

52. Walk one to three miles daily

53. Learn to lift properly

54. Throw away your tie

55. Make sure your receive proper dental care

56. Use a mini trampoline

57. Do flexibility exercises

58. Live as close to your work as possible

59. Don't smoke

60. Don't drink alcoholic beverages

61. Choose a good mattress and a neck-conforming pillow

62. Don't sleep on your stomach

63. Take a hot bath daily

64. Drink filtered water

65. Bathe in filtered water

66. Do your best to avoid doctors

67. Keep the bowels regular

68. Learn all you can about health and wellness

Be happy

69. Have a positive attitude

70. Laugh a lot

71. Share enthusiasm

72. Develop a strong and abiding faith

73. Work to build a happy marriage

74. Pursue at least one hobby

75. Make sure yours is a purpose-driven life

76. Help others

77. Follow a career or occupation you enjoy

78. Keep pets and enjoy them

79. Make sure you get what you expect

80. Practice yoga

81. Reduce the stress in your life

82. Always be faithful to your spouse

83. Tell the truth so you won't have to remember your lies

84. Do a good deed every day of your life

85. Shun credit cards

86. Be friendly and helpful to your neighbors

87. Avoid anger

88. Learn something new every year

89. Read good books

90. Stay away from all forms of pornography

91. Don't take yourself too dammed seriously

92. Listen to good music

93. Enjoy your children and grandchildren

94. Get involved with sports that you can play all of your life

95. Keep smiling

96. Learn to play bridge and other games that require you to think and remember

97. Socialize with other people in your church and neighborhood

98. Be the best you can be

99. Join a service club and volunteer for club projects

100. Keep the romance in your marriage

101. Be of service to your fellow man

102. Have a good sex life

103. Hug as many people as you can each day without getting into trouble

104. Look for the good in everyone

105. Don't gossip

106. Compliment as many people as you can each day

107. Attend the church or synagogue of your choice regularly

108. Read your Bible or other book of faith regularly

109. Be forever grateful

110. Never criticize, condemn, or complain

111. Don't tell people your troubles. Eighty percent don't care and the other twenty percent are glad you're having trouble

112. Keep the same schedule every day

Simple rules to help you control your weight

- Avoiding white sugar, white flour, salt, and all soft drinks, including diet drinks

- Eating only whole grain products

- Preferring fresh over frozen, and frozen over canned foods

- Purchasing organic foods whenever possible

- Eating most of your food in the raw state.

- Eating meat sparingly after all fat has been trimmed off. The white meat of chicken and turkey with the skinned trimmed off are the best. Don't undercook meat because of the risk of salmonella or trichinosis and don't charcoal it because of the increased threat of cancer.

- Choosing cruciferous veggies such as cauliflower and broccoli.

- Not drinking fruit juices. They are loaded with calories and fructose or fruit sugar. A glass of orange juice has 180 calories and turns to sugar in a very short time whereas one orange has sixty calories, is more filling and because of the fiber takes an hour to raise your blood sugar.

- Including an ounce of almonds, pecans, or walnuts per day to provide you with essential fatty acids.

- Cooking your food in canola or olive oil and avoiding all cooking fats that contain trans-fatty acids.

- Drinking half an ounce of water a day for every pound of body weight and even more during hot weather or when you perspire a lot.

- Avoiding tea, except for green tea, coffee, alcohol, sodas, or milk, except for skim milk.

● Liquids should be drunk at least one hour before meals and one-half hour after meals to prevent the weakening of your digestive juices.

● Eating slowly, chewing each bite as thoroughly as possible and not reading or watching TV during your meals.

● Eating small meals every few hours to keep your blood sugar at the proper level.

● Not eating late at night or snacking late in the evening except perhaps for a piece of fruit.

Winning over high blood pressure

More than ninety medications have been developed to treat high blood pressure. They have one thing in common: serious side effects including death, impotency, muscle deterioration, and more.

One wonders how the treating physician makes a decision about which of the ninety remedies for high blood pressure to prescribe.

Blood pressure medications could probably be avoided in more than half of all high blood pressure cases by following a few simples rules:

1. Lose weight and keep your weight under control.

2. Exercise daily. A walk of one to three miles will reduce your blood pressure by twenty millimeters.

3. Magnesium reduces high blood pressure with the only side effect that it may increase the number of bowel movements per day.

4. Biofeedback is effective in reducing blood pressure. Sitting in a chair, letting all your muscles relax, and picturing calming scenery in your mind will do much to lower your blood pressure.

5. Avoid squabbles and confrontations with employees, friends, and relatives.

6. Drink an adequate amount of liquid.

7. Avoid caffeinated drinks.

8. Avoid whole milk. Use skim milk instead.

9. Follow a fat-free diet.

10. Prefer fruits and vegetables plus whole grain cereals.

11. Use a good salt substitute and stop using salt.

12. Take garlic and fish oils.

Ten Commandments for Longevity

If you want to live to be 100 I would suggest that you follow my Ten Commandments for Longevity.

1. **Diet.** Eat lots of fruits, vegetables, and whole grains. Raw, organic foods are best for you. Fresh better than frozen, frozen better than canned is the rule.

2. **Vitamins and minerals.** Absolutely essential for longevity. For every dollar you spend on vitamins you save many dollars in health care expense.

3. **Exercise.** Many diseases can be prevented or cured by exercise. It improves your circulation, prevents and controls diabetes, prevents constipation, increases lung capacity, and makes you look younger.

4. **Sleep.** Seven to nine hours is best. More sleep indicates your body is worn out. Too little sleep will wear you out faster. A noon nap is worth an hour's sleep at night.

5. **Attitude.** A negative attitude towards life will shorten your life and may actually make you sick.

6. **Laughter.** Laughter increases the endorphins in your body helping your immune system. Most comedians (Bob Hope, George Burns are examples) live a long life.

7. **Church.** Statistics show that people who attend church live an average of seven years longer than non-churched people.

8. Marriage. A good marriage to the right person also increases your life expectancy by seven years.

9. Massage. Good for relieving tension and releasing toxins from your body. Excellent even for babies.

10. Chiropractic adjustments. When your spine's in line, you'll feel fine.

Benefits of exercise

There are few health care protocols that offer such inexpensive benefits as regular exercise. Those benefits include the following:

1. Reduces the risk of heart disease.

2. Improves circulation.

3. Reduces and prevents obesity.

4. Lowers LDL cholesterol.

5. Raises HDL cholesterol.

6. Increases the vital capacity of the lungs.

7. Prevents diabetes and helps control blood sugar levels.

8. Lowers blood pressure in the hypertensive patient.

9. Raises blood pressure for the low blood pressure patient.

10. Reduces stress.

12. Prevents depression.

13. Prevents osteoporosis by increasing bone density.

14. Improves the immune response of the patient.

15. Improves muscle tone.

16. Suppresses appetite when done before a meal.

17. Improves mental outlook on life.

Sugar: 76 Ways Sugar Can Ruin Your Health

The following article is reprinted with the permission of Nancy Appleton, Ph.D, from her book, *Lick The Sugar Habit* (www.nancyappleton.com). Sugar may cause the following diseases or health problems—

- Sugar can suppress your immune system and impair your defenses against infectious disease.

- Sugar upsets the mineral relationships in your body: causes chromium and copper deficiencies and interferes with absorption of calcium and magnesium.

- Sugar can cause a rapid rise of adrenaline, hyperactivity, anxiety, difficulty concentrating, and crankiness in children.

- Sugar can produce a significant rise in total cholesterol, triglycerides and bad cholesterol and a decrease in good cholesterol.

- Sugar causes a loss of tissue elasticity and function.

- Sugar feeds cancer cells and has been connected with the development of cancer of the breast, ovaries, prostate, rectum, pancreas, biliary tract, lung, gallbladder and stomach.

- Sugar can increase fasting levels of glucose and can cause reactive hypoglycemia.

- Sugar can weaken eyesight.

- Sugar can cause many problems with the gastrointestinal tract including: an acidic digestive tract, indigestion, malabsorption in patients with functional bowel disease, increased risk of Crohn's disease, and ulcerative colitis.

- Sugar can cause premature aging.

- Sugar can lead to alcoholism.

- Sugar can cause your saliva to become acidic, cause tooth decay and periodontal disease.

- Sugar contributes to obesity.

- Sugar can cause autoimmune diseases such as: arthritis, asthma, multiple sclerosis.

- Sugar greatly assists the uncontrolled growth of Candida Albicans (yeast infections)

- Sugar can cause gallstones.

- Sugar can cause appendicitis.

- Sugar can cause hemorrhoids.

- Sugar can cause varicose veins.

- Sugar can elevate glucose and insulin responses in oral contraceptive users.

- Sugar can contribute to osteoporosis.

- Sugar can cause a decrease in your insulin sensitivity thereby causing an abnormally high insulin levels and eventually diabetes.

- Sugar can lower your Vitamin E levels.

- Sugar can increase your systolic blood pressure.

- Sugar can cause drowsiness and decreased activity in children.

- High sugar intake increases advanced glycation end products (AGEs) (Sugar molecules attaching to and thereby damaging proteins in the body).

- Sugar can interfere with your absorption of protein.

- Sugar causes food allergies.

- Sugar can cause toxemia during pregnancy.

- Sugar can contribute to eczema in children.

- Sugar can cause atherosclerosis and cardiovascular disease.

- Sugar can impair the structure of your DNA.

- Sugar can change the structure of protein and cause a permanent alteration of the way the proteins act in your body.

- Sugar can make your skin age by changing the structure of collagen.

- Sugar can cause cataracts and nearsightedness.

- Sugar can cause emphysema.

- High sugar intake can impair the physiological homeostasis of many systems in your body.

- Sugar lowers the ability of enzymes to function.

- Sugar intake is higher in people with Parkinson's disease.

- Sugar can increase the size of your liver by making your liver cells divide and it can increase the amount of liver fat.

- Sugar can increase kidney size and produce pathological changes in the kidney such as the formation of kidney stones.

- Sugar can damage your pancreas.

- Sugar can increase your body's fluid retention.

- Sugar is enemy #1 of your bowel movement.

- Sugar can compromise the lining of your capillaries.

- Sugar can make your tendons more brittle.

- Sugar can cause headaches, including migraines.

- Sugar can reduce the learning capacity, adversely affect school children's grades and cause learning disorders.

- Sugar can cause an increase in delta, alpha, and theta brain waves which can alter your mind's ability to think clearly.

- Sugar can cause depression.

- Sugar can increase your risk of gout.

- Sugar can increase your risk of Alzheimer's disease.

- Sugar can cause hormonal imbalances such as: increasing estrogen in men, exacerbating PMS, and decreasing growth hormone.

- Sugar can lead to dizziness.

- Diets high in sugar will increase free radicals and oxidative stress.

- High sucrose diets of subjects with peripheral vascular disease significantly increases platelet adhesion.

- High sugar consumption of pregnant adolescents can lead to substantial decrease in gestation duration and is associated with a twofold increased risk for delivering a small-for-gestational-age (SGA) infant.

- Sugar is an addictive substance.

- Sugar can be intoxicating, similar to alcohol.

- Sugar given to premature babies can affect the amount of carbon dioxide they produce.

- Decrease in sugar intake can increase emotional stability.

- Your body changes sugar into 2 to 5 times more fat in the bloodstream than it does starch.

- The rapid absorption of sugar promotes excessive food intake in obese subjects.

- Sugar can worsen the symptoms of children with attention deficit hyperactivity disorder (ADHD).

- Sugar adversely affects urinary electrolyte composition.

- Sugar can slow down the ability of your adrenal glands to function.

- Sugar has the potential of inducing abnormal metabolic processes in a normal healthy individual and to promote chronic degenerative diseases.

- IVs (intravenous feedings) of sugar water can cut off oxygen to your brain.

- Sugar increased the risk of polio during the polio epidemic.

- High sugar intake can cause epileptic seizures.

- Sugar causes high blood pressure in obese people.

- In intensive care units: Limiting sugar saves lives.

- Sugar may induce cell death.

- In juvenile rehabilitation camps, when children were put on a low sugar diet, there was a 44 percent drop in antisocial behavior.

- Sugar dehydrates newborns.

- Sugar can cause gum disease.

The above article is scientifically referenced.
For more information on problems associated with sugar, go to www.mercola.com/article/sugar/dangers_of_sugar.htm.

A word about chiropractic

A leader in wellness

The chiropractic profession is a leader in matters pertaining to wellness. Understanding the musculoskeletal system and spinal health is one of our outstanding contributions made to health care.

In May 2000, *Consumer Reports* reported that a survey of 46,000 people showed that for back pain 35 percent used alternative therapies, including chiropractic. Chiropractic received more positive responses such as "helped me feel better" than any other form of care. In 1994, the U.S. government-published guidelines for the Agency for Healthcare Policy and Research shows that spinal manipulation for lower back pain is safe and effective for both pain management and improving functionality.

The Magna Report funded by the Ontario Ministry of Health in Canada states, "For the management of low back pain chiropractic care is the most effective treatment, and it should be fully integrated into the government's health care system."

A study showed that chiropractic care was more effective than hospital outpatient management mainly for chronic or severe lower back problems. Chiropractic patients were three times more satisfied with their care than patients of Family Practice Physicians.

Chiropractic care of a variety of neuromusculoskeletal conditions is gaining wider acceptance in society. Medical referrals to doctors of chiropractic particularly for back pain are increasing rapidly. Approximately 89 percent of conditions cared for by chiropractors relate to the musculoskeletal system which comprises sixty percent of all body systems.

An article in *Spine Journal* designated spinal manipulation at generally accepted, well established, and widely used. A majority of family physicians in the state of Washington admitted to having encouraged patients to seek chiropractors and two out of three indicated a desire to learn more about what chiropractors do.

Chiropractic is one of the largest health care professions in the United States and is the fastest growing primary health care profession in the world. There are more than 65,000 active licenses for doctors of chiropractic in the United States and 8,000 students currently studying chiropractic curriculum.

In the United States there are three Healing Arts licenses to provide health care. They are traditional medicine, chiropractic, and osteopathy. Chiropractic health care is included in federal programs such as Medicare, Medicaid, the Government's Employee Hospital Association Benefit Plans, and thousands of insurance programs. Chiropractors now serve important parts of the health care in numerous Armed Services health care facilities.

Sixty million people seek chiropractic care each year. The *Journal of American Medical Association* affirms that Americans are more likely to visit a non-medical provider than a medical doctor. Expenditures associated with alternate therapy amounted to a fraction of the cost of medical care.

Chiropractic subluxations or misalignments are thought to stimulate neuroreflexes. Every organ and tissue in your body is influenced in some way directly or indirectly by the nervous system. Any dysfunction of one system may have far reaching and significant effects on the nervous system. William Boyd, MD, with his classic work, *A Textbook of Pathology*, states that disease, whether the heart, kidneys, or brain is disturbed function, not merely a disturbed disordered structure.

Chiropractors follow a conservative approach and do not use prescription drugs or surgery. The chiropractic approach endeavors to establish and maintain normal body function by correcting spinal and other joint misalignments. Chiropractors believe that health comes from within your body from inside out rather than from the outside in as is the common practice with drugs or with surgery to remove a diseased organ.

Most headaches are not caused by a deficiency of aspirin but rather a subluxated vertebra in the neck. Have you ever noticed when you have a headache you twist your neck in different positions and massage your neck?

If every organ and tissue cell in your body is controlled by nerves, you need to normalize the nervous system by gentle spinal adjustments.

Chiropractors start treatment with a thorough case history and examination, take X-rays if necessary, and then try to correct the misalignments to restore normal function.

You hear a lot of great things about chiropractors.

Lance Armstrong is featured in a recent issue of *Esquire Magazine.* He is shown receiving a chiropractic adjustment. During his marathon Tour de France races, a mobile chiropractic unit traveled with him so that he could get daily chiropractic care.

Mel Gibson, the producer of *The Passion of Christ,* lists his chiropractor in the credits following the movie. The Wrangler Rodeos use chiropractors to treat the tremendous trauma sustained by the bull and horseback riders. Most National Football League teams have chiropractors taking care of the numerous neuromusculoskeletal problems of their players.

President Eisenhower when he traveled on his train campaigning for election had a chiropractor accompany him on the train. President Truman walked to his chiropractor's office every week after his presidential career was ended. Arnold Schwartzanegger's best man at his wedding was his chiropractor.

Dr. Phil recently stated on his show that he visits his chiropractor regularly. Arnold Palmer was in a golf tournament several years ago and asked for a chiropractor to help him because of his stiff neck. He received care and proceeded to win the tournament. Barry Bonds has a contract with the San Francisco team that wherever he goes to play they must have a chiropractor to adjust him before he swings his bat.

The Veterans' Administration recently passed a regulation providing chiropractic care as a benefit to veterans. Chiropractors are now commissioned in the Armed Services.

Chiropractic has come along way since I graduated fifty-two years ago. At that time, very few insurance companies paid for chiropractic services. Now most insurance companies pay for chiropractic services. Medical doctors used to be vitriolic in their condemnation of patients that went to chiropractors. Now many referrals to chiropractors are made by medical doctors.

Half a century ago the public was told that there was no such thing as a pinched nerve. Now after CT Scans, MRI, and other specific scientific equipment, doctors representing all specialties are realizing the importance of pinched nerves.

Chris Carter of the Minnesota Vikings team said the most important man on the team was his chiropractor and his massage therapist. Tiger Woods represented the chiropractic profession on the Rose Parade centennial float in 1995.

You do not have to be famous to benefit from chiropractic services. Remember, only a chiropractor can determine whether or not you are a chiropractic patient.

The chiropractic paradigm

The paradigm of chiropractic care is predicated on the fact that your nervous system either directly or indirectly controls every function of the body. You cannot swallow, digest, absorb, or eliminate without the supervision of the nervous system. You cannot sit, stand, walk, run, blink, or reproduce without the nervous system being involved.

The spinal column protects the spinal cord, which contains thirty-one branches of nerve fibers emitting on either side of the spinal cord and eventually terminating in the tiny tissue cells. It is imperative for a normal transmission of nerve impulses from the brain to the tissues to take place.

The brain is the super computer that runs the body through the nervous system. Minute nerves like electrical wires run from the brain inside the spine, branching out in thirty-one pairs of nerve fibers. These nerves lead to all of the organs and tissues of your body. The brain is responsible for homeostasis, the physiological balance of all your organs and tissues for your benefit.

Misalignments and subluxations of the spine result from trauma, stress, and poor posture. Chiropractic care consists of the removal of nerve interference in order to bring about the normal expression of nerve function. Instead of relying on a proper diagnosis for recovery, the chiropractor is concerned about finding the subluxations and pinched nerves within the spine and then correcting the misalignments so that normal function takes place.

Think about it! Is your headache caused by a deficiency of aspirin or Tylenol? Is your ulcer caused by a deficiency of Maalox? Is your constipation a shortage of ExLax in your body?

The goal of medicine is either to stimulate a lack of function of the body or inhibit an excessive function of the body. Chiropractic care is designed to normalize all the functions of all of the organs and tissues in the body.

Many famous athletes find it to their advantage to have regular chiropractic care. Tiger Woods, Lance Armstrong, Joe Montana, Martina Navaratala, Ivan Lendel, Billy Jean King, Barry Bonds, and others have been quoted in the news media giving chiropractic credit for getting them back on the playing surface.

The entire USA Women's Volleyball Team had chiropractic adjustments the night before they won the World Championship. The careers of many athletes have been extended as a result of chiropractic care.

Remember, when your spine's in line, you'll feel fine. If you have a spine, you need a chiropractor. Chiropractic care will benefit the whole family. My children received their first adjustment on their way home from the hospital after their birth.

My Views on Chiropractic

by Rev. George Boyajian

Editor's note: This article was written in the mid-1950s. Rev. Boyajian came to Davenport on a stretcher; more dead than alive, and through the chiropractic care he received at the Palmer Chiropractic College clinics regained his health and proclaimed the benefits of chiropractic.

A magnetic healer comes in contact with a colored janitor who has been deaf for 17 years. In a shouting conversation he learns that his hearing loss occurred after he had stooped under some steps to clean and something popped in his neck.

While examining Harvey Lillard's neck he notices a bump or swelling on the side of his neck. The magnetic healer reasons that if the bump caused the deafness, the reduction of such would restore the hearing. He gives the janitor a thrust in the neck, the janitor's hearing is restored, and thus in that seemingly chance occurrence is born the science of Chiropractic, which has been a blessing to millions of ill people, and will, I chance to prophesy, be still a greater blessing to ever increasing multitudes in the days that lie ahead.

During the course of my ministry I was taken quite ill, and inasmuch as I realized that my health had failed considerably, I sought the best medical help available in the east. In the course of a visit to the doctor's office, I informed him that among other difficulties I was suffering from insomnia at night and severe exhaustion during the day. He reached for his prescription pad and in well nigh undecipherable semi-Latin hieroglyphics prescribed two kinds of medication, Phenobarbital for the insomnia and Benzedrine Sulfate for the exhaustion.

Being possessed of an inquisitive type of mind, I decided to ask a pharmacist friend what reactions these drugs were intended to produce in the system. I was informed that Phenobarbital was a sedative and Benzedrine sulfate a stimulant. To my utter amazement I was taking both a sedative and stimulant during the course of the same day! I am sure the reader realizes that one need not possess a brilliant mind to see the utter paradox and absurdity of such a procedure. To me, in the sphere of the healing arts this was illogic at its very height. And it may be said without hesitancy that whosoever breaks logic, logic breaks him. Then and there I determined that my ill body was not to be the experimental situation on which this broken logic was to be tried.

It was not long before I came to the conclusion that if medicine knew the cause of disease it would not have to resort to such contradictorily methods of approach. Medicine was essentially dealing in the realm of the province of effects and not causes: that by the use of medication it was simply shutting off Nature's warning signals (symptoms) that something was wrong within. To shut off the fire alarm while the house is burning does not put out the fire. It simply fails to give notice that the conflagration is taking placed. To block symptoms while failing to give heed to what caused the symptoms would not get at the basis of the difficulty. The end thereof of such an approach would be nothing short of further breakdown in health.

Having come thus far in my thinking, I purposed to read the attitudes of eminent medical authorities on the subject of medicine and disease. I discovered some very interesting statements and attitudes expressed by leading men of the twentieth century in the fields of medicine and surgery.

Sir William Osler, famed founder of Johns Hopkins Medical School in Baltimore Maryland, said that to interfere with Nature's efforts to heal disease costs too much money, too much time, too much in suffering, and prolongation of illness, far too much on the whole, for Nature knows how to cure disease but man does not, and "anything that could not be cured by Nature must forever remain uncured." Voltaire said. "We put medicine, of which we know little, into bodies about which we know less to cure disease of which we know nothing at all." Osler further stated that he could count on the finger of one hand without repeating, all of the so-called remedies that are of any use to the human race. Not long before he died he said, "The cause of disease is still a great mystery."

The late Dr. Charles Mayo of the famed Mayo Clinic of Rochester, Minnesota, said at an open meeting of the American College of Surgeon quite a few years ago: "Nine-tenths of the internal surgery that is done today should never have been done, and the seemingly necessary tenth part should be done by someone who has some further evidence of surgical ability than merely a diploma in medicine."

Rev. Boyijean sought the services of an Osteopath, a Naturopath, an Allopath, and began to wonder if all "paths" led to the grave.

At the suggestion of a friend Rev. Boyijean finally consulted a chiropractor, was referred to the Palmer College Research Clinic. He completely recovered from his many maladies and became one of chiropractic's most articulate spokespersons.

People who have used chiropractic with great success

These famous people and 50,000,000 others have benefited from chiropractic care.	
John D. Rockefeller	Arnold Palmer
President Dwight Eisenhower	Phyllis Diller
Eleanor Roosevelt	President Harry Truman
Joe Montana	Charles Malone
Billy Jean King	Jason Sasser
Stan Smith	Erin Brachovich
Fred Cox	Lance Armstrong
Jerry Rice	Rev. Robert Schuller Jr.
Roger Craig	The World Champion Women's Soccer Team
Ted Danson	Tiger Woods
Bob Cummings	Mel Gibson
Emmett Smith	Lance Armstrong
Hubert Humphrey	Mary Lou Retton

You don't have to be rich or famous to benefit from chiropractic care. Every year millions of people all over the world trust their health to doctors of chiropractic usually after all else has failed.

On August 16, 2001 Erin Brachovich told the Washington Press Club that her chiropractor was responsible for her life story being written and made into a movie for which Julia Roberts won the Academy Award for her performance.

In a sports page I read a story about Viking receiver superstar and NFL record holder Chris Carter. This football hero gives credit not to his team mates but to his chiropractor, massage therapist and trainer for his success on the field. Carter has never missed a game and has led the team in receptions for the last eight years.

Lance Armstrong, Tiger Woods, the entire championship women's soccer team, the St. Louis Rams and Cardinals, Joe Montana, Jerry Rice, Carl Lewis and many other championship teams and individual superstars have relied on chiropractic care to help prevent and heal their injuries.

Chiropractors have a hundred-year history of treating athletes quickly and effectively, many times avoiding spine, shoulder, elbow, knee, and ankle surgeries.

Joe Montana was recently described by John Madden as the greatest quarterback that ever played football. After he was severely injured by a tackle that causes a ruptured disc, surgery was performed. Many thought that his career was ended. However, thanks to chiropractic care he was back playing just eight weeks later. He went on to win several Super Bowl rings and set many NFL records.

When the Forty-Niners played Denver in the Super Bowl in Florida, Joe was interviewed on national television while getting an adjustment before the game. It was questionable whether Jerry Rice, who had injured an ankle the week before, would be able to play. Chiropractor Nick Athens was flown to Florida to adjust Jerry's ankle. Not only was he able to play; he was the Most Valuable Player of the game. Dr. Athens adjusted thirty-three Forty-Niners before the game. San Francisco won 55 to 10.

Barry Bonds set the home run record with 73 during 2001. Bonds has a contract that calls for a chiropractor to be present at the clubhouse locker room to adjust him before every game. Most national sports teams now have chiropractors taking care of their athletes. Dan O'Brien, gold metal winner in the decathlon, recently told an audience of 7,000 people in Las Vegas that his medical doctor told him he would have to quit running because of his bad back. Several visits to a chiropractor corrected his back problem and enhanced his physical performance. O'Brien said he planned to enter the next Olympics at 38 years of age.

Tiger Woods, Emmitt Smith, and Chris Carter are just a few other athletes that have publicly endorsed chiropractic care for correcting their injuries and enhancing their skills.

Notes from the Palmer College 100th Anniversary

Dr. B. J. Palmer, the developer of chiropractic, printed cards one hundred years ago stating "Keep Smiling" on the reverse side of his professional card. At a recent observation of the anniversary of Dr. Palmer's contribution to health and healing, I noted the following comments.

W. B. Clark, M.D.: There was never a time where over ten percent of the world's population was ever vaccinated for smallpox.

George Bernard Shaw: "More people die from vaccinations than the disease they were designed to prevent."

- Every single vaccine can cause encephalitis.
- One percent of vaccinated kids wind up with autism.
- Vaccines contain aluminum, mercury, and formaldehyde.
- Your body is a whole lot smarter than your doctor.
- The U.S. is the most vaccinated country in the world and we are one of the sickest nations.
- Only one in fifty vaccine damaged children is reported.
- Crib deaths were unheard of before vaccination became mandated.
- Bubonic plague, typhoid fever, tuberculosis, and scarlet fever disappeared without vaccines.
- Vaccines are not studied in combinations.
- A five-pound child and a sixty-pound child may receive the same dosage.
- Interference and damage to the nervous system may seriously damage your immune system.
- You were born to be healthy.
- Forty-five vaccines by age six, seventy-four before graduating from high school.

- Health care profits from disease, not from health.
- Psychiatric drugs have tripled since 1991.
- Medical doctors are great for treating trauma and eye disorders.
- Medicine is both expensive and dangerous.
- Symptoms are a message.
- Forty percent of the time the first symptom of a heart attack is death.
- Seventy-five trillion cells in the human body. Two hundred thousand chemical reactions are taking place per second.
- The universe is organized. Organization=intelligence
- Hanging analogy; disconnects the brain from the body.
- Are you interested in a Life Doctor or a Disease Doctor?
- Dr. Towbin found in 1969 ninety percent of crib deaths had neurological damage.
- Dr. Gutman studied two thousand newborns and found that seventy-five percent of newborns had neurological damage caused by delivery.
- Eighty pounds of pressure may be exerted on the head and neck of a newborn.
- Fifty percent of children are dropped during their first two years of life.
- Subluxations affect more people than any other condition known to man.
- We have seen a fifteen percent annual increase in the marketing of drugs during the last several years.
- Forty million people see a chiropractor every year.

Choosing chiropractic as a career

Eddie Crandall was one of the best employees that ever worked for the Hagen Chiropractic Clinics.

Eddie's husband was president of the Student Activities Committee of Sioux Falls College. He had been injured in a severe car accident several years earlier. During hospitalization after the accident, his medical doctors advised him never to go to chiropractors. R.J. checked himself out of the hospital and made an appointment to see a chiropractor who was receiving excellent results. He responded well to treatment. While working at the Hagen Clinics, Eddie advised her husband to have some X-rays made and seek care for the migraine headaches caused by the whiplash accident, and a series of several adjustments ensued. Excellent results were achieved. After graduating, R.J. worked full-time with the Boy Scouts of America in the Sioux Falls area.

I decided to encourage R.J. to consider chiropractic as a career. One problem he faced was that his four years of college were in the humanities and the prerequisites for chiropractic studies required six hours of biology, six hours of chemistry and six hours of physics. Therefore he had to complete another year of college before enrolling at the Palmer College of Chiropractic in Davenport, Iowa.

One day Eddie observed a totally disabled patient who was able to walk immediately after an adjustment by Dr. Hagen. This incident was the impetus she needed to convince R.J. to become a chiropractor. Her brother Mike had written a ten-page report on chiropractic during his high school studies. Both R.J. and Mike are now Doctors of Chiropractic and have built a new clinic in Beatrice, Nebraska.

Eddie received her degree in Wellness from Sioux Falls College and ran the Rehabilitation Programs at the Hagen Clinic in Sioux Falls.

Eddie's mother, a registered X-ray technician, worked in their clinic and Eddie's father built their outstanding chiropractic clinic. Eddie commented on a recent visit how pleased she was with the delivery of her four children and the general health of her children thanks to chiropractic adjustments. We felt vindicated further by a Chicago area medical doctor who testified against the AMA several years ago in a court case, stating that women under chiropractic care during their pregnancies delivered in half the time that women who had not received chiropractic adjustments required.

She worked with patients supervising exercise programs to strengthen their muscles and ligaments to speed up their recovery. She was delighted to use the entire lower level, which was furnished with special rehabilitation equipment, to work with her patients.

My oldest patient

Not long ago I lost my oldest patient. She was 105 years of age. I had taken care of her for forty years. She came to me for every ache and pain that she had. Her husband and daughter were killed in a car accident. She survived but had fractured her spine and broken her hip. Her frequent chiropractic care kept her working in a restaurant until she was in her 80s. I kidded her that on her 100th birthday she would get a free adjustment, and she got that adjustment.

She lived alone and took care of herself until she was 102, and then as she was going to sit on a bench in her garden, she missed the bench and fractured her pelvis. She wound up in a nursing home. I would occasionally see her when I journeyed into northwest Iowa.

Last year, we lost her. She did not die of disease. She did not die of old age. She was in a chair that would assist her in getting up and down out of the chair, and the chair malfunctioned and threw her forward on her face. She died of the injuries. She was sound of mind and, had it not been for her recent fracture of the pelvis, sound of body as well. She was a delight to take care of.

I went to her 100th birthday party expecting to see about a dozen of her friends. There were 180 people at her birthday party. She looked younger than her daughter. My wife was astounded to see this vivacious lady at 100 years of age in such command of her physical and mental well being.

Adjustments save asthma victim's life

I was attending the Clay County Fair at Spencer, Iowa. A vendor selling agriculture equipment called me over. "Do you remember me?" he asked.

"No," I said, "I don't."

"When I was an infant I suffered from severe asthmatic attacks. The medical doctors advised my parents I would not live very much longer. My parents called you, and you came out to our home and adjusted me on an ironing board." He no longer suffers from asthma.

That reminded me of another child patient that I adjusted on an ironing board. Ludwig Hansen, a native of Germany, lived across the street from us. One day their daughter fell off the davenport and went into convulsions. The medical doctor was called and demanded she be hospitalized and put on anti-convulsive medications. Ludwig refused. I was called. She also was adjusted on an ironing board; she never had another seizure.

Will the author live to be 100?

My goal in life is to be the last survivor of World War II. I am a 24-day veteran of World War II.

Will I live to be 100? I doubt it. Unfortunately, for the first fifty years of my life, I did not eat judiciously. For many years I consumed a pint of ice cream almost every day. After attending a Nathan Pritikin seminar for doctors around the world, I cleaned up my bad eating habits and lost forty pounds. I've maintained my proper weight for years.

As I've mentioned already, I've never missed a day of work. I went over fifty years without taking an aspirin. I've never had an ibuprofen product or tried Viagra. Since I turned fifty, I have taken a lot of vitamins, and I exercise daily—especially in the wintertime.

So why can't I live to be 100? Anything is possible, but I was run over by a trailer when I was six years old, and a stallion stepped on the middle of my back. I have ruptured six discs in my spine due to whiplash, over lifting, and the stallion incident. I also landed on the pavement after falling off a bicycle to keep from hitting a pickup truck and had the nose wheel collapse on my airplane during take-off.

All of these mishaps and mistakes took a toll on my body and will probably shorten my life. Then there's the genetic factor. I don't know of anyone in my immediate family line who lived to be 100.

Does that mean I should give up living healthfully? Of course not. Whether I have one year or thirty left to live, I want to be as strong and healthy as I possibly can be. I could be hit by a dump truck tomorrow, and that's all the more reason for living a healthy life today. Join me!

Appendix

Vitamin and mineral deficiencies caused by various substances

Alcohol: Vitamins A, D, E, K, B_1, B_2, B_3, B_5 (pantothenic acid), B_6, B_{12}, C, biotin, choline, folic acid, inositol, and PABA. Mineral deficiencies of calcium, cobalt, magnesium, plus problems with carbohydrate and fat metabolism may occur.

Antacids: Vitamins A, D, B_1, B_5 (pantothenic acid), B_{12}, bioflavinoids, and folic acid. calcium, cobalt, iron, and phosphate depletion may occur.

Caffeine: Vitamins A, B_1, B_2, B_3, B_{12}, B_{15}, bioflavinoids, biotin, choline, folic acid, inositol, and PABA. Mineral depletion includes calcium, chloride, cobalt, iron, magnesium, potassium, and zinc. Water is also affected by the diuretic effect of caffeine.

Antibiotics: Vitamins K, B_2, B_3, B_5 (pantothenic acid), B_6, B_{12}, C, biotin, choline, folic acid, and PABA. Mineral depletion may include calcium, cobalt, magnesium, potassium, and zinc.

Aspirin: Vitamins K, B_1, B_{12}, C, bioflavinoids, and folic acid.

Birth control pills: Vitamins E, B_1, B_2, B_6, B_{12}, C, bioflavinoids, and folic acid. The minerals calcium, cobalt, copper, iron, and magnesium are interfered with.

Cholesterol drugs: The fat-soluble Vitamins A, D, E, and K.

Cola drinks: Vitamins K, B_6, B_{12}, biotin, choline, folic acid, and PABA. The minerals calcium and cobalt, and other water soluble vitamins.

Diuretics: All of the water soluble Vitamins (B complexes and Vitamin C). The minerals calcium, chloride, magnesium, potassium. Water is also lost as the result of the ingestion of diuretics.

Estrogen: B_2, B_6, B_{12}, biotin, choline, folic acid, and PABA. The minerals calcium and cobalt are depleted.

Laxatives: The fat soluble vitamins A, D, E, and K, plus B_1, B_{12}, C, and the bioflavinoids. The minerals calcium, cobalt, copper and potassium are diminished.

Smoking: Vitamins A, D, B_1, B_2, B_3, B_5 (pantothenic acid), B_6, B_{12}, C, the bioflavinoids, biotin, and folic acid. The minerals calcium, cobalt, and copper are negatively affected by smoking.

Steroids: Vitamins A, D, B_6, C, and the bioflavinoids. The minerals calcium, potassium, selenium, and zinc are depleted.

Stress: Vitamins A, E, B_1, B_3, B_5 (pantothenic acid), B_6, B_{12}, C, the bioflavinoids, and biotin. The minerals calcium, potassium, plus water are reduced by stress.

Sugar: Vitamins B_1, B_2, B_3, and C. The minerals calcium, chromium, magnesium, phosphorous, potassium plus interference with carbohydrate and fat metabolism.

Recommended reading

Confessions of a Medical Heretic by Robert Mendelson, MD

Male Practice by Robert Mendelson, MD

How to Raise a Healthy Child in Spite of Your Doctor, Robert Mendelson, MD

The Essential Guide to Prescription Drugs 2004 by James J. Rybacki, Pharm.D.

Death by Medicine by Gary Null, Ph.D.

The Complete Encyclopedia of Natural Healing by Gary Null, Ph.D.

Bottom Line Year Book 2006 by the editors of Bottom Line Personal

Nutritional Chart by Dr. Bruce Hagen

Depletions Chart by Dr. Bruce Hagen

Prescription for Nutritional Healing by Dr. James and Phyllis Balch

The Womanly Art of Breast Feeding by Gwen Gotsch and Judy Torgus

The Medicine Men by Leonard Tushnet, M.D.

Modem Medical Mistakes by Edward Lambert, M.D.

The Medical Racket by Martin L. Gross

The Doctors by Martin L. Gross

The Drug Story by Morris Beale

Natural Cures They Don't Want You to Know About by Kevin Trudeau

A Stolen Life by Marge Grant (Her son suffered irreparable vaccine damage), www.dptshot.com

Malignant Medicine by Joel Kaufman, Ph.D.

Statin Drugs Side Effects by Duane Graveline, M.D., Ph.D.

Recommended subscriptions

Alternatives by Dr. David Williams,
www.drdavidwilliams.com

Bottom Line by Bottom Line Publishers

The Dr. Julian Whitaker Newsletter, www.drwhitaker.com

The Dr. Stephen Sinatra Newsletter, www.drsinatra.com

Mercola.com free e-mail newsletter, www.mercola.com

The Blaylock Wellness Report, www.newsmax.com/
blaylock

Dr. Ted Korens newsletter and articles,
www.korenpublications.com

Curriculum Vitae: Bruce C. Hagen

Dr. Bruce C. Hagen grew up in Southern Wisconsin. Born at home, he saw a medical doctor twice before graduating from high school. He enlisted in the US Army Air Corps upon graduation the week of his seventeenth birthday. While in the Air Force he served in Texas, Guam, and Japan where he attended Keio University, and Fort Cambell, KY.

He attended the Palmer College of Chiropractic in Davenport, Iowa and interned with Dr. R. A. Silbaugh, a professor at Palmer College in Wheatland, Iowa. He received a BAS degree from Westmar College in LeMars, Iowa. He received a Certificate of Management from the American Management Association at Morningside College in Sioux City, Iowa. Additional studies include "The Latest Strategies in Treating Low Back and Sciatic Nerve Disorders" at the Harvard School of Medicine in Boston, "Managing Physicians," "Health Systems Management," "Industrial Ergonomics," "The Latest Strategies in Health Systems Management," and "Negotiating Health Care Contracts," all of which were conducted at the Harvard School of Public Health, and seminars, including Carpal Tunnel at the Stritch School of Medicine, Loyola University; Acupuncture, x-ray, Industrial Consulting, Athletic Injuries, and Nutritional Evaluation.

Dr. Hagen is the author of numerous articles and books on health including "Clinical Procedures and Patient Management," "Practice Administration," "The Personal Injury Practice, the largest nutritional chart ever published, "Depletions Chart" and a genealogical book entitled, "From Whence Came I?" He has lectured to chiropractors from every state in the Union and several foreign countries.

Dr. Hagen continues to practice with his son Dr. Mark Palmer Hagen at one of the nations finest chiropractic clinics in Sioux Falls, South Dakota. Both doctors are team chiropractors for the Sioux Falls Canaries baseball team and the Sioux Falls Sky Force professional basketball teams. He and his wife Beth have presented free chiropractic clinics in Jamaica five times, once in the Ukraine, and five times in Poland where they have given over a million dollars in free services, clothing, and health care items.

His professional address is Hagen Chiropractic Clinic, 3405 S. Kiwanis Ave., Sioux Falls, SD 57105, 605-361-0UCH.

Website: DRBRUCEHAGEN.COM